FAMILY MEDICINE AND PRIMARY CARE

Jan De Maeseneer

FAMILY MEDICINE AND PRIMARY CARE

At the Crossroads of Societal Change

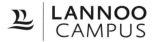

For Anita

D/2017/45/304 – ISBN 978 94 014 4446 0 – NUR 870

Cover design: Paul Verrept
Interior design: theSWitch
Artwork cover: Interrelated Connectedness by Guy Timmerman | © Photo: Studio Claerhout

LannooCampus Publishers is a subsidiary of Lannoo Publishers,
the book and multimedia division of Lannoo Publishers nv.

LannooCampus Publishers
Erasme Ruelensvest 179 box 101
3001 Leuven
Belgium
www.lannoocampus.com

Content

Foreword

Family medicine and primary health care made major advances since the Alma-Ata Declaration of the World Health Organisation (WHO) in 1978.[1] What was initially seen as a sound principle – to structure health care from the community level in response to the needs of individuals and populations – turned out to be a determining factor of effective, efficient, safe and timely health care.[2] With WHO's reconfirmation of primary health care as the core component of health systems in the World Health Report of 2008,[3] the international development of primary health care with a central role for Family Medicine within it truly got under way. This book reviews and critically appraises these developments.

The 40 years since 'Alma-Ata' largely overlap with the history of the World Organisation of Family Doctors (WONCA), which was founded in 1972. Over time, a strong alliance has grown between WHO and WONCA to support the restructuring of health systems from hospital-centric to community-based.[4] This is still very much a work in progress, with few formal evaluations to date. This book, based on the author's impressive international track record, comes at an important time, as reflective personal experiences and observations are very valuable contributions. The excitement of international primary health care development is in applying the general principles of caring for all individuals for all health problems at all life stages, while integrating prevention, promotion of health, care and support in a person- and population-centred approach over time and in a way that adapts to the local context. The local community is a core determinant of the final outcome of this process of change. In its ten chapters this book covers the various aspects of primary health care development – from regulating the health system to the teaching and education of (future) primary health care professionals.

The importance of this book should be seen in the light of two fundamental lessons that have been learned from international primary health care development. First, the process of changing from hospital- to community-based health systems is challenging and requires coherent policies. It has to address regulatory issues such as how to ensure access to health care and the affordability of health care. It also involves defining indicators that allow measurement of the process of system change over time. This process of change requires close collaboration with community leaders, academics, health funders, health professionals and other stakeholders. Consistent policy is required, in which all the various aspects are addressed as interrelated components. Changing the health structure without training adequate numbers of health professionals with the skills and competencies to practice in the primary health care setting, or providing specialty training without a regulated role for family physicians in the health system, will substantially hamper the performance and ongoing development of the health system, and the capacity to provide universal health coverage.

Secondly, primary care and family medicine are highly complex fields. The successful development and implementation of policy require that this complexity is understood and respected. The impact of primary care and family medicine is not just in the process of health care, but in the outcome through improvements in the health status of individuals and communities, their functioning, and autonomy. What people can do themselves should not be taken over by professionals. Interventions should not be provided just because of their availability, but only when they contribute to people's health status. When the provision of disease-specific interventions is replaced by responsiveness to individual and community needs, the orientation of care can be directed at and evaluated in terms of individually specified goals.

The essence of the professionalism and effectiveness of family medicine is in understanding individuals and communities and sustaining trusted relationships with these constituencies. Professional concepts go well beyond the traditional medical reference of diseases and interventions, as is true for the markers of quality primary health care. In the end it is always back to the basics: the person, family, and local community. Social conditions are the main determinants of health and disease, and even within close geographic proximity, communities may substantially differ in their social conditions.[5] A major contribution of primary care to population health and well-being is in including this awareness in the health care provided to individuals.

The 40 years since Alma-Ata, and the organisational life history of WONCA, span also the professional and academic career of the distinguished author of this book, Professor Jan De Maeseneer, our colleague and friend. Jan not only lived through this period, but has been a creative maestro orchestrating the development of primary care and family medicine as a global movement.[6] The ten chapters of this book represent the various domains where Jan has made his academic mark. This book testifies to his leadership. At the same time it is a monument to his many magnificent contributions. There is no better way for the international community of primary health care to commemorate his farewell from the Chair of Family Medicine and Primary Health Care at Ghent University.

Professor Amanda Howe, President of WONCA 2016-2018
Professor Michael Kidd, President of WONCA 2013-2016
Professor Rich Roberts, President of WONCA 2010-2013
Professor Chris van Weel, President of WONCA 2007-2010

Introduction

This book tells the story of family medicine and primary care, as I have experienced it, explored it, learned it, practised it, taught it, changed it and – to some extent – also lived it. The first chapter describes the journey of the 65 years behind us. In the following chapters topics as varied as social determinants of health, Goal-Oriented Care, making a diagnosis, the social accountability of pharmaceutical industry, the care for quality, the organisation of primary care, physician payment systems and global primary care are discussed. Each chapter starts with a "(patient-)story" and ends with a reflection from an expert in the field. The chapters are co-authored by (former) staff members of the Department of Family Medicine and Primary Health Care at Ghent University. However, I take full responsibility for the content of this book.

The chapters are built on a mix of scientific facts and subjective perceptions of someone who was actively involved and tried to make change happen.

Although in some continents there are important differences between general practitioners (meaning someone with only basic undergraduate medical training in most African countries), in this book we use "family physicians" and "general practitioners" interchangeably, both indicating a professional specifically trained to fulfil a comprehensive medical function in primary care.

The final chapter looks at the way forward, exploring why nowadays, more than ever, the world needs strong primary care.

This book wants to contribute to the reflection on how to create societies based on social cohesion, focusing on what really matters: peace, connectedness, compassion, solidarity, social justice, truth and hope for a sustainable future for all.

Jan De Maeseneer

Chapter 1:

A Personal View on the History of Family Medicine and Primary Care

I knew Ann-Mary for many years in the practice. She visited regularly for neck pain, sometimes she had worries about the two children growing up, she worked in a bank, played tennis, and was what one could call "an exemplary patient". On a Monday morning in March 2000, she visited me with a story of increasing pain situated somewhere around the stomach, but radiating to the back. Her anxiety and the information that "this was a different type of pain than what she was used to", alerted me, and I referred her for immediate medical imaging. Two hours later, she came back, and the diagnosis was clear but at the same time devastating: "Stomach cancer, already involving the liver and the diaphragm". The following eight months were filled with hope and despair, but most of all were marked by her courage. The oncologist, the resident, the nurse, we all participated in her journey, from surgery over chemotherapy, and finally the decision to go for a palliative approach. The interaction with her husband and children, looking at the past, dealing with the present and already preparing for the future, made us the privileged partners in what human beings are able to cope with, to share, to fear and to celebrate.

Ann-Mary took the lead and organised the care. She had the courage to testify in front of the students what this disease meant to her and her family, creating one of those moments that shapes the students' future profile as physicians.

And then she decided to stop therapy, because it did not help, and to choose "quality of life". Ann-Mary appreciated everything that made her life comfortable and was grateful for the days she could enjoy with her family. Between Christmas and New Year, she died peacefully at home in the arms of her husband and children.

Her husband recently reminded me of this painful episode: "We still miss Ann-Mary so much!"

I Was Born on 30 June 1952

I was born on 30 June 1952 in a local hospital in the city of Ghent in Belgium, the second child in a family that later had 6 children, and contributed consistently to the "baby boom" of the fifties. The study career of my parents ended at the age of 14-16 years, as the Second World War started. They married after the war. My father had a job at a newspaper, where he gradually became the deputy general director, and my mother stayed at home, to take care of the children. Our parents gave us the opportunities they did not receive themselves and enabled us to go to secondary school and to university. We all graduated at Ghent University.

It is noteworthy that in 1952 the delivery was performed by the family physician and a midwife, illustrating the comprehensiveness of the discipline of family medicine in those days. Family doctors were male and took care of the individuals and families they all knew very well "from the cradle to the grave". They mainly provided reactive care, responding to the dominant disease pattern: acute (infectious) conditions like influenza, pneumonia, sinusitis,... Family physicians had an in-depth knowledge of families and were consulted for a lot more than "biomedical diseases". Doctors had to advice on what school the children had to go to, on whether it was a good idea to move to another building, they were asked for advice in case of job loss,... Counselling about "family planning" was another in those days new task, but not an easy enterprise, as a family physician reported; *"Oh yes! There was the contraceptive pill. But we, doctors, were very conservative and in the beginning we thought the contraceptive pill is unnatural. When I graduated in 1960, our professor of gynaecology told us that there was a medication to regulate irregular menstruation and 'maybe you could prescribe that in exceptional cases, when it is really indicated to use this for some sort of family planning*[7]*'. The first patient who asked for the contraceptive pill I refused the prescription, but finally, we had to accept it"*. Family physicians acted at "the crossroads of societal change" during that period, probably one of the most important changes in the twentieth century!

Family Medicine and Primary Care

At the Same Time in the United Kingdom: Development of General Practice (GP)

In the United Kingdom (England) Collings described the development of general practice in the fifties.[8] He started his article as follows: "General medical practice is a unique social phenomenon. The general practitioner enjoys more prestige and wields more power than any other citizen, unless it be the judge on his bench. In a world of ever-increasing management, the powers of even the senior manager are petty compared with the powers of the doctor to influence the physical, psychological and economic destiny of other people... General practice is unique in other ways also. For example, it is accepted as being something specific, without anyone knowing what it really is. There are no real standards for general practice. What a doctor does, and how he does it, depends almost wholly on his own consigns". And then follows a "grim analysis of present position and future prospects". But the recommendations are positive: "First, an attempt should be made to define the future province and function of general practice within the framework of the National Health Service. Secondly, basic group-practice units should be formed as soon as possible. There is real urgency about launching this experimental work; for relatively soon the new patterns of hospital and specialist care will be firmly established, and everything will be fitted into them. If that happens it will then be virtually impossible to do very much about general practice".

The concept of "primary care" also originated from the United Kingdom. Already in 1920 Lord Bertrand Dawson proposed three hierarchical levels of "care location" (primary, secondary, tertiary). He first identified "primary care as the most basic level of a structured health system, concerned with caring for common problems in outpatient settings".[9]

In the Netherlands the fifties saw a strong development of general practice/family medicine. At the start in October 1956, the Dutch College of Family Medicine decided to organise the famous Woudschoten-Conference, that finally led to the definition of the function of the family physician: "To accept the responsibility for a continuous, integrated and personal care for the health of individuals and families, which they are accountable for. This care focuses on the prevention when possible and a cure of disturbances in the health status of the individual and the family (a threefold task: to cure, to rehabilitate and to prevent)".[10] It is amazing to see how "modern" the vision of some of the participants at that conference was. So was the vision of Buma, who described an "anthropological diagnosis": the description of somatic issues, an analysis of the psycho-functional situation, and an "ecological description". Querido[11] sees the patient as a person integrating the somatic, the social and the psychological field. Comprehensive care does not mean that the physician should address everything on his own, but that he should deliver care in co-operation with social workers, psychiatrists and mental health professionals. Finally, the Woudschoten-Conference defined 12 tasks for the family doctor (see box 1).

Box 1. Tasks of the family doctor, according to the Woudschoten-Conference

1. Primary care in the broader sense, including addressing psychological traumata.
2. Somatic examination.
3. Psychological and ecological examination that requires appropriate skills in communication and history taking.
4. Registration and management of all medical data.
5. Differentiation in 2 approaches: one group that can be approached according to daily routine, and a group that requires specific approaches because of the complexity of the problems.
6. Treating what the family physician is able to address.
7. Task delegation to medical and other providers, but with maintenance of the co-responsibility.
8. Making a plan for follow-up in concordance with the medical specialists involved and taking care of its execution.
9. Integration and co-ordination of the care for the patient, for the disabled by appropriate co-operation with other providers.
10. Contributing to prevention.
11. Contributing to health promotion and education.
12. Continuous professional development recognising the possibilities and limitations.

Countries like the United Kingdom, Denmark and the Netherlands took two measures that helped the discipline of family medicine to develop: the organisation of care based on a "patient list system" and a "gatekeeping" mechanism, meaning that patients could not access a specialist doctor without a referral letter by the family physician. In Belgium and France these conditions were not fulfilled, which led in the 1960's to a progressive "erosion" of the discipline of family medicine, because the developing technology and the possibilities for interventions in hospitals confirmed Collings' warnings.

In absence of a sound scientific underpinning family physicians worked "experience driven", exploiting the opportunities of the strong personal relationship with individuals and families which provided them with a lot of "contextual evidence". Increasingly, family physicians addressed psycho-social problems, inspired by new developments like the "antipsychiatry"-movement and the ideas of Thomas Szasz, as developed in the *Myth of Mental Illness* (1960) and *The Manufacturer of Madness: a Comparative Study of Inquisition and the Mental Health Movement* (1970), emphasising the right to self-determination and questioning the medical metaphors that label behavioural disturbances as "diseases".

May '68... and Dreaming about a Community Health Centre

I was studying at the secondary school when May 1968 marked the student movement in Berkeley, Paris,... Books like Herbert Marcuse's *One-Dimensional Man: Studies in the Ideology of Advanced Industrial Society* (1964) criticised consumerism, arguing that it is a form of social control and that the system we live in may claim to be democratic, but is actually authoritarian in that view that individuals dictate our perceptions of freedom by only allowing us choices to buy for happiness. This results in a "one-dimensional" universe of thought and behaviour in which aptitude and ability for critical and oppositional behaviour wither away. One of the ideas formulated in this book was "The Great Refusal", when Marcuse makes clear that individuals must develop a new radical subjectivity, so as to create the conditions for social transformation: The Great Refusal is fundamentally political, a refusal of repression and injustice, a saying no, a noncompliance with the rules of a rigid game, a form of radical resistance and struggle.

The ideas of the "tiers-mondistes" like Frantz Fanon and Helder Camara brought the global perspective to students' actions. Most inspiring were teachers in the secondary school who started innovative ways of teaching: small group work, using what happens in society as the starting point of an educational reflective process,... Student participation in secondary school was one of the landmarks in the movement towards "democratisation" of the school and I became the president of the "Students' Council" at our school. The role models by teachers, as well as the "student movement" bringing all secondary schools in the city of Ghent together, in order to change content of curricula and make it more relevant to understand the societal challenges, was very inspiring. Paul Heirwegh, our Latin teacher, stimulated me to explore in my final "maturity exam" historical evolutions in an essay comparing "imperialism" in the Roman Empire as described in "Ab Urbe Condita" by Titus Livius (1st Century BC) with the work of Helder Camara, an advocate of liberation theology, fighting for the poor and for Human Rights and democracy during the military regime (Brazil – 20th Century). Theoretical concepts were put into practice through fund-raising for the support of liberation movements in developing countries, like Frelimo in Mozambique, SWAPO in Namibia, MPLA in Angola and ANC in South-Africa. All these experiences shaped my world view in those days.

When I started to study civil engineering in 1970, it soon became clear that this could not be my future. I tried to share issues on social justice, human rights with fellow engineer students, but they were not interested. The "hidden curriculum" did not stimulate critical thinking and the study load was huge.

Contacts with students who were active in the follow-up of the May 68-movement in the Faculty of Medicine and who looked for innovation and change in health care delivery, inspired my choice to shift to the studies in medicine. To be honest, I started to study medicine with the aim to change the health care system. But during medical training I discovered that I loved to take care of patients and to address health problems.

From the first medical year onwards we organised a "Social Working Party", looking at social determinants of health and how it affects the health of migrants, prisoners, unemployed people,... Later on, we started the "MORDICUS-student working party", looking at how we could change the curriculum (organising "alternative lectures" debating the need for a new professionalism and more "social justice" in health), but also engaging in reflection on a new perspective for the profession of medicine.

In the framework of a project of educational innovation in the undergraduate programme at Ghent University, under the leadership of Professor Karel Vuylsteek (Social Medicine), groups of students had to analyse a relevant problem that could make a difference in health and society. Our group was working on the topic of "Community Health Centres" and published a report in 1974 where we proposed that "A community health centre is a co-operation of different health care providers (nurses, family physicians, social workers, physiotherapists,...) working together on an equitable basis as far as function, impact on policy and financial reward is concerned. The aim is to realise a comprehensive (psycho-socio-somatic) care of people living in a neighbourhood focusing on health literacy and empowerment, in order to contribute to a health care system, involving the population of the neighbourhood in the governance. We defined a neighbourhood as a group of people with similar interests and needs living in the same geographical area". This concept of Community Health Centres was inspired by experiments such as the "Local Centre for Community Health: Pointe-Saint-Charles" in Montreal (Canada), by primary health care centres in the United Kingdom and in the Netherlands. In follow-up of this document, interprofessional working parties started to reflect with students in nursing, medicine, physiotherapy and social work on how a Community Health Centre could offer an innovative perspective for professionals in health care.

Friday 24 September 1976: medical students occupy Ministry of Health

In the seventies, there was no formal training for family medicine in Belgium. In 1975, the conservative medical trade unions, under the leadership of Dr A. Wynen (in those days president of the World Medical Association), proposed a "revalorisation of family physicians", through an increase with 20% of the fee-for-service tariffs for family doctors who had followed one hundred hours of "additional education". The regulation stipulated that the family doctors only had to follow these one hundred hours once, and then they would be allowed to increase their tariffs for the rest of their career. For the organisation of Dr Wynen, this was a strategy to enlarge his organisation, that mainly consisted of specialist doctors, with family physicians. But that was not the end of the story: he also developed the idea of a post-graduate training for "specialist-family physicians" that would become the 26th "speciality" in medicine in Belgium. By doing so, the "family physicians" would become one of the specialties and the ongoing debate about a gatekeeping role for the family doctor could be stopped. The idea was that the trade unions of doctors would organise the post-graduate training for family doctors themselves, consolidating their influence on the training of specialist doctors with a new track for family physicians. The Minister of Health decided to put the debate on the agenda of the High Council for Specialist-Doctors, where the position of the organisation of Dr Wynen was dominant.

The students did not agree at all with this development. Already in March 1976, there was a manifestation by medical students in Brussels, where they asked for an improvement of the 7 years undergraduate training, before a debate about post-graduate training could be considered. Moreover, the plans for the post-graduate training were that 50% of the training would take place in hospitals, that were in need of "cheap labour". The students opposed to the idea that there would be 2 types of family physicians: one with low-tariffs (without any additional training) and one with "higher tariffs".

In September 1976, a document on "Specific criteria for the training and recognition of family physicians who want a special qualification in the framework of the National Institute for Health and Disability Insurance: NIHDI" (meaning: the right to access higher tariffs), was published.

The students could not agree with the document, especially because there was only 6 months training in family medicine labelled as: "The trainee will help a preceptor in family medicine during 6 months".

In order to stop the process, the students of all the medical faculties in Belgium decided to occupy the meeting room of the High Council of Specialists that would debate the proposal on the 24th of September 1976.

At 6 p.m., the 50 delegates of the High Council of Specialists that were supposed to meet were sitting in the meeting room in the centre of Brussels, when all of a sudden 150 to 200 medical students entered the room preventing the meeting and clearly formulating the viewpoints they had agreed upon. I was one of the spokesmen of the students and our action made clear that we wanted a serious debate about the quality of the undergraduate training, the need for an appropriate post-graduate training in family medicine and the need for a transformation of the High Council for Specialist Doctors towards a "High Council for Family Physicians and Specialist Doctors".

The message of the students also reached the academic world, and in Flanders, 8 years later, an interuniversity training with strong academic input and a high level of participation by the students was developed (see Chapter 7). Medical students have actively participated in the societal debate about the future of medicine and health care ever since.

New Inspirations for Family Medicine

In *Medical Nemesis: The Expropriation of Health*,[12] published in 1975, Illich challenged the practice of medicine, blaming it for "clinical iatrogenesis" (the fact that there are a lot of side effects and hospitalisations due to medical intervention and therapies), for "social iatrogenesis" looking at the "medicalisation of life" and the fact that increasingly care was transferred from the contexts where people lived to institutions, and finally for "cultural iatrogenesis" indicating that people were no longer able to give meaning in their life to pain, disease and death. This provocative work offered a fundamental reflection on the way health care was developing in the seventies, and created an opportunity for family medicine and primary care to really find their place especially when it comes to "putting people at the centre of the care process". In 1976 I had the privilege to participate in a seminar at Ghent University, where Illich translated his analysis into a strategy for change. I was fundamentally impressed by his vision, by the sharpness of his analysis, and his relentless search for using the correct formulation when exploring a problem.

Also in 1976 Byrne and Long focused on the process of doctor-patient communication. They distinguished 6 phases which form a logical structure to the consultation: the doctor establishes a relationship with the patient; the doctor either attempts to discover or actually discovers the reason for the patient's attendance; the doctor conducts a verbal or physical examination or both; the doctor or the doctor and the patient, or the patient (in that order of probability) consider the condition; the doctor, and occasionally the patient details further treatment or further investigation; the consultation is put to an end, usually by the doctor. Byrne and Long also analysed the range of verbal behaviours doctors used when talking to their patients. They described a spectrum ranging from a heavily doctor-dominated consultation with any contribution from the patient basically excluded, to a virtual monologue by the patient untrammelled by any input from the doctor. Between these extremes, they described a gradation of styles from closed information-gathering to non-directive counselling, depending on whether the doctor was more interested in developing his own line of thought or the patient's.[13]

In 1977 Engel published his article on the bio-psycho-social model, indicating that the psychological and social aspects had been overlooked in the biomedical model, whilst they are an important component of "being ill". Behaviour and environment are of utmost importance in the genesis, the development and the experience of illness. And disease or being ill also influences the psychological well-being and social relationships.[14]

This insight was also very much emphasised by Ian MacWhinney in his approach to family medicine in Canada. Ian MacWhinney moved to North America in the late sixties and family medicine in Canada was just getting on its feet, it was redeveloping, re-emerging as a distinct discipline. MacWhinney observed:

"I thought that it was strange and wrong that the biggest branch of medicine, in terms of numbers of positions, had no representative in medical school. So what kind of medicine would students learn?".

There was a rush to specialisation and the idea was that everybody would need a cardiologist, a gerontologist and an obstetrician, and MacWhinney enunciated the fact that there was a specialty, a body of knowledge, a scientific basis for taking care of people in their lives. *"This means that as well as classifying the patient's illness, giving it a name, which is still of course crucial, that we also don't feel that we've finished our task until we know what the illness means to the patient"*, MacWhinney said. He is without doubt the single most influential individual in the development of the discipline of family medicine upon which the Canadian health care system depends. He established the intellectual basis for it, and began with the first training program in the discipline in Canada.

All these developments were very positive, but in some countries, especially in those where more and more parts of care had been transferred from family medicine to specialist care, the increasing interest in the psycho-social domain was a kind of "compensation" for the diminishing impact in the biomedical field and became reason for concern. Some family physicians started "specialising" in "psychotherapy", leaving the "generalist" field behind.

1978: Alma-Ata Declaration

1978 was the year of the Alma-Ata Declaration on Primary Health Care. Professor Karel Vuylsteek attended this important meeting of the World Health Organisation in Kazakhstan. In those days he was involved (with Professor André De Schaepdrijver and others) in the preparation of a Department of Family Medicine and Primary Health Care at the Faculty of Medicine at Ghent University.[15] So, he brought a very inspiring message: broadening the scope of Primary Health Care could contribute to "Health for All". When re-reading the Declaration today, one is amazed by the relevance of the concepts and the pertinence of the strategies that were described in this document (see box 2).[1]

Box 2: Alma-Ata Declaration, Chapter VI and VII

VI.
Primary health care is essential health care based on practical, scientifically sound and socially acceptable methods and technology made universally accessible to individuals and families in the community through their full participation and at a cost that the community and country can afford to maintain at every stage of their development in the spirit of self-reliance and self-determination. It forms an integral part both of the country's health system, of which it is the central function and main focus, and of the overall social and economic development of the community. It is the first level of contact of individuals, the family and community with the

---

national health system bringing health care as close as possible to where people live and work, and constitutes the first element of a continuing health care process.

VII.
Primary health care:

1. reflects and evolves from the economic conditions and sociocultural and political characteristics of the country and its communities and is based on the application of the relevant results of social, biomedical and health services research and public health experience;
2. addresses the main health problems in the community, providing promotive, preventive, curative and rehabilitative services accordingly;
3. includes at least: education concerning prevailing health problems and the methods of preventing and controlling them; promotion of food supply and proper nutrition; an adequate supply of safe water and basic sanitation; maternal and child health care, including family planning; immunisation against the major infectious diseases; prevention and control of locally endemic diseases; appropriate treatment of common diseases and injuries; and provision of essential drugs;
4. involves, in addition to the health sector, all related sectors and aspects of national and community development, in particular agriculture, animal husbandry, food, industry, education, housing, public works, communications and other sectors; and demands the co-ordinated efforts of all those sectors;
5. requires and promotes maximum community and individual self-reliance and participation in the planning, organisation, operation and control of primary health care, making fullest use of local, national and other available resources; and to this end develops through appropriate education the ability of communities to participate;
6. should be sustained by integrated, functional and mutually supportive referral systems, leading to the progressive improvement of comprehensive health care for all, and giving priority to those most in need;
7. relies, at local and referral levels, on health workers, including physicians, nurses, midwives, auxiliaries and community workers as applicable, as well as traditional practitioners as needed, suitably trained socially and technically to work as a health team and to respond to the expressed health needs of the community.

The most important factor determining the success of Alma-Ata Conference was that it brought up the issue of the right of every human being and every nation to health care and health promotion, to a new, global level, under the new historical conditions. The important factor in determining the success was the recognition of the primary health care philosophy. This involves the fact that the health of the population is linked to the social and economic development of society. Another factor was the conclusion pertaining to developing countries:[16] the conference demonstrated that even the poorest countries could do something to help themselves and not simply wait for help from outside.

Selective Primary Health Care

Shortly after its publication the Alma-Ata Declaration was criticised for being too broad and idealistic and having an unrealistic time table, especially in the slogan "Health for All by 2000". In 1979 the Rockefeller Foundation sponsored a conference "Health and Population in Development" in Bellagio (Italy). Important stakeholders attended the meeting, e.g. Robert S. McNamara, President of the World Bank. He promoted business management methods and clear sets of goals, advocating poverty reduction approaches. The conference discussed the paper "Selective Primary Health Care, an Interim Strategy for Disease Control in Developing Countries".[17] In that paper a strategy based on "basic health services" was presented. Selective primary health care was introduced as the name of the new perspective. The term meant a package of low-cost technical interventions to tackle the main disease problems of poor countries. These interventions were summarised in the acronym GOBI-FFF (Growth monitoring, Oral rehydration techniques, Breast-feeding, Immunisation, Food supplementation, Female literacy, Family planning). Selective primary health care quickly attracted the support of donors, scholars, and agencies.

A debate between the two versions of primary health care was inevitable: on the one hand comprehensive primary health care, on the other hand selective primary health care.[18] The supporters of comprehensive primary health care accused selective primary health care of being a narrow techno-centric approach that diverted attention away from basic health and socio-economic development, did not address the social causes of disease and supported vertical programs. Newell formulated his critic as follows: "[Selective primary health care] is a threat and can be thought of as a counterrevolution. Rather than an alternative, it can be destructive. Its attractions to the professionals and to funding agencies and governments looking for short-term calls are very apparent. It has to be rejected".[19] Moreover, the new political context characterised by the emergence of conservative neo-liberal regimes in the main industrialised countries drastically reduced the funding for health care in developing countries. There was also an issue in acceptance of primary care by health professionals: very often they perceived primary health care as anti-intellectual, promoting pragmatic non-scientific solutions and demanding too many self-sacrifices. The resistance of medical professionals increased, as they feared to lose privileges, prestige and power.

In 1988 the election of Nakajima as WHO director-general, succeeding the charismatic Halfdan Mahler, the "father" of the Alma-Ata Declaration, marked the end of the first period of primary health care. It was only in 2008, with the World Health Report "Primary Health Care: Now More Than Ever!", that a new era for primary health care started. Even now, the debate between selective primary health care and comprehensive primary health is still ongoing, and transferring funds from vertical disease-oriented programs to strengthen primary health care, remains a challenge.[6]

Starting as a Family Physician and Developing a Community Health Centre

In 1977, after my graduation as medical doctor, my wife Anita De Winter and I stayed in Rwanda for 3 months (Africa). Anita finalised the clerkships of her last medical year, whilst I was working at the Community Health Centre in Gisagara as a volunteer. This experience was an eye opener: working in a Community Health Centre, looking at the health needs of a population, investing in health promotion and empowerment, providing cure and care, made the theoretical concepts more operational and demonstrated how such an approach could make a difference. The struggle to find intersectoral strategies to save lives of undernourished children (kwashiorkor, marasmus) brought the inspiration for what later would become the Community Health Centre in Ledeberg (Ghent-Belgium).

In 1978, Anita and I started a practice in Ledeberg, a deprived area of the city of Ghent. It started as a simple practice with family physicians, operating in the fee-for-service system and offering primary health care. Anita worked during 11 years in the practice and then decided to become a psychiatrist, working in secondary care, both in ambulatory setting and in hospital.

Very soon the practice turned into an interprofessional group practice (with nurses, social workers, dieticians) and finally in 1981 into an interprofessional Community Health Centre "Botermarkt". We started different projects: developing integrated interprofessional home care, including palliative care at home; developing health promotion at the community level; organising group sessions for pregnant women (and their partners); organising group sessions on "relaxation",.... The health status of many patients was poor, with a lot of addiction problems, unhealthy behaviour (alcohol, smoking, lack of physical activity,...). During the home visits, we observed unhealthy living conditions with low quality of the housing. As the neighbourhood of Ledeberg had become part of the bigger city of Ghent in 1977, almost all welfare agencies, including the Public Centre for Social Welfare, had left the neighbourhood for more "centrally located" premises. As the needs were high, any project that was started by the Community Health Centre, was well received, and there was no competition with other agencies at all. The Community Health Centre tried to look at the "bigger picture" and to tackle the "upstream causes" of the health problems. So actions were developed to improve housing conditions.

On Thursday 1 September 1983 we were confronted with an accident where a young pedestrian was severely wounded when crossing the street in front of the Community Health Centre, leading to an action on traffic safety (Chapter 8). Another intervention was related to the lack of green spaces in the neighbourhood causing a level of physical activity of the youngsters that was far below the average in the Flemish region. In all these actions there was an intensive participation by different stakeholders in the neighbourhood (youth organisations, organisations of the elderly, local police, care providers, schools,...). Although we were not aware of the concept, we later discovered that the strategy we used was actually Community Oriented Primary Care[20] (see chapter 2).

From the very beginning we looked for a financing mechanism that was more appropriate than fee-for-service with co-payment (up to 33%), in order to help us achieve the goal of accessible Integrated Person- and People-Centred Care, with a strong emphasis on prevention and health promotion. With other Community Health Centres in Belgium, we first tried to mobilise politicians for a new law, installing a system of salary-financing of health care providers in Community Health Centres. Unfortunately, the proposal was never debated in parliament. So, we changed strategy and revitalised an article in the basic law on health insurance that had almost never been used, but created the possibility to develop a capitation system in an interprofessional primary care setting (see Chapter 9). In 1982 the negotiations with the health insurance companies (in the framework of the National Institute for Health and Disability Insurance NIHDI) ended with an agreement that enabled the development of an integrated flat-rate capitation system for family medicine, nursing and physiotherapy, based on the average reimbursement per person in the fee-for-service system. However, as computers were not yet available in the health care system, it took a long period to overcome the administrative burden and finally on 1 April 1995 Community Health Centre "Botermarkt" started in the capitation-system with 1700 patients on the list, that grew to 6200 today (2017). Importantly there was no co-payment for the patient in this capitation system.

In 1986, after an intensive preparation by the social worker, we started a platform on "Caring for the Community", bringing all the stakeholders of primary care in the neighbourhood together to meet regularly and to discuss the problems in the neighbourhood, trying to formulate a "Community Diagnosis". Apart from representatives of the local population, including representatives of the youth, the elderly, ethnical cultural minorities,... all primary care providers participated, together with public health agencies (for children, for school health,...), social work, home care organisations, local police, schools, community workers,... This platform is actually transformed into the "Network: Society-Welfare-Health" focusing on active participation of all stakeholders and intersectoral action for health. The advantage of such a network is that individual providers can send "signals" to the network members about problems in the care process, and if the problem cannot be resolved at the community level, it will be transferred to the City Health Council. When needed it could even go to the regional or federal Ministry of Health.

The developments in the Community Health Centre were strongly inspired by the "Ottawa Charter for Health Promotion" that was launched by WHO in 1986. The Ottawa Charter defined health promotion as "The process of enabling people to increase control over, and to improve their health. To reach a state of complete physical, mental and social well-being, an individual or group must be able to identify and to realise aspirations, to satisfy needs, and to change or cope with the environment. Health, therefore, is seen as a resource for everyday life, not the objective of living. Health is a positive concept emphasising social and personal resources, as well as physical capacities. Therefore, health promotion is not just the responsibility of the health sector, but goes beyond healthy lifestyles to well-being".[21] The insights of this charter were translated in the community of Ledeberg in a project "Working together for health", that involved Ghent University, the city of Ghent, different stakeholders in the community,... and received support from the Council of Europe.

Becoming an Academic, Involved in Health Policy Development

Whilst practising part-time as a family doctor in the Community Health Centre Botermarkt in Ledeberg, I started to work at the new Department of Family Medicine that was inaugurated at the Faculty of Medicine of Ghent University in October 1980, under the leadership of Professor René De Smet. We started with a team of 3: Professor René De Smet, myself as a half-time assistant, and a part-time secretary. The task was huge: to develop both undergraduate and postgraduate teaching in family medicine, to start research, to recruit a staff of active family physicians with an interest in academic work. René De Smet chose most of the group of practising family physicians from the new generation of young practitioners that were interested in developing new ways of organising care: group practices, multidisciplinary co-operation, networks, CHCs,... In 1984, the four departments of family medicine in Flanders decided to work together for one integrated postgraduate training program. This co-operation has contributed a lot to the strengthening of family medicine and primary health care (in Flanders), not only in the field of teaching, but also in the field of research and policy development (see Chapter 7).

In 1984, inspired by the work of the "WONCA International Classification Committee" (the Classification Committee of the World Organisation of Family Doctors), that developed the "International Classification of Primary Care"[22] (ICPC), I started a registration project in over one hundred family practices, collecting data (with paper and pencil as computers were not yet available) of 5609 family physician-patient encounters that were coded using ICPC. This data collection was the basis for my PhD thesis, the first that was made in Belgium in the field of Family Medicine. However, in 1975 Professor Jan Heyrman (KU Leuven) was the first Flemish family physician to obtain a PhD title in Utrecht (the Netherlands) with a project on developing a screening tool for good nutrition habits.

Apart from an epidemiological description, my PhD thesis analysed the relationship between the functioning of family doctors and the problems they were dealing with, looking at their problem-solving strategies and the correlation between performance and attitudes. One of the conclusions of my PhD research was that the more "defensive" the attitude of the family physicians was (always preferring the certain to the uncertain), the more laboratory tests they ordered, the more they referred patients to specialists e.g. in case of cardiovascular problems, the more they prescribed antibiotics in case of respiratory problems and benzodiazepines in case of psycho-social problems.[23] Another important finding of the research was that workload of family physicians matters: family doctors who see more than 30 patients a day are less patient-centred in their communication and prescribe more drugs per diagnosis. In analysing the functioning of family doctors, we used 4 clusters of variables: doctor-, diagnosis-, patient- and encounter-characteristics. Especially when it comes to the analysis of prescription of medicines, this "multi-level" approach is of utmost importance. This first PhD thesis examining the family physician-patient interaction at the consultation level in Belgium, triggered a lot of debate in the country. Immediately after the public defence, the federal Minister of Health and Social Affairs, Philippe Busquin, asked me to become his advisor for primary health care. My first project for the minister was to set up a mechanism where patients could subscribe to a patient list of a family physician who took the responsibility to integrate all information (from hospital, from nursing, from social work,...) in the "Global Medical Record" of the patient. Although there was a double mechanism to stimulate this process (on the one hand the doctor was paid annually a lump sum per patient to update the Global Medical Record, on the other hand the patient who subscribed to a list obtained a higher reimbursement for consultations and home visits with the practice that kept his/her Global Medical Record), it took lots of debates and 12 years of implementation before the whole population had access to this mechanism in 2002. Now more than 70% of the Flemish population has a Global Medical Record with a family medicine practice.

Head of Department of Family Medicine and Primary Health Care at Ghent University

In 1991 I was appointed as Head of Department of Family Medicine and Primary Health Care by the Faculty of Medicine of Ghent University. When looking for relevant papers to underpin the teaching of the frameworks of family medicine and primary health care at the department, we came across the paper on "Goal-Oriented Medical Care" by James Mold from the University of Oklahoma[24] (see Chapter 3). Mold made a clear plea to shift the medical practice from a disease orientation towards an orientation focusing on the patient's goals in terms of quantity and quality of life. We immediately integrated this seminal paper into our course on family medicine and primary health care in the undergraduate medical curriculum. These ideas were further developed, but it was only in 2011 that we were able to start research on this paradigm shift in interaction with teams in Oklahoma, Maastricht University in the Netherlands and the University of Western Ontario (Canada). Perhaps one of the reasons that "Goal-Oriented Care" did not break through widely, was that in 1992 Gordon Guyatt and his colleagues published another landmark paper: "Evidence-Based Medicine", an important paradigm shift in the approach to the practice of medicine.[25] In the beginning, certainly public health and family medicine were the disciplines that took the lead in the development of "evidence" and the translation of this evidence into "guidelines" that fundamentally reshaped the practice. "Evidence-Based Medicine" brought family medicine in many countries back in the field of "clinical medical care" and contributed a lot to the revival of the discipline. In 1996, David Sackett and colleagues warned us that Evidence-Based Medicine is not a "cookbook" approach, and that it is important that patient values are integrated into Clinical Decision Making.[26] This indirectly underpinned the importance of Goal-Oriented Care.

Nowadays, in different countries, thousands of guidelines have been developed based on evidence. This has fundamentally changed the practice of family medicine and has become a corner stone in quality assurance, not only within the discipline, but also in the framework of interprofessional co-operation. However, there was also a danger in using the "evidence" in a reductionist way, changing the goal of "treating the patient" to "treat-to-target". The way the pharmaceutical industry has tried to "integrate" evidence in promotional campaigns, has contributed a lot to this reductionism (see Chapter 5). In 2003 in a paper in The Lancet[27] we argued that apart from "medical (or better: professional) evidence" there is a need for "contextual evidence" and also "policy evidence", in order to achieve improvement in the quality of care (see Chapter 6).

Family Medicine Goes Global

During the last decade of the 20th century the discipline of family medicine spread to regions like Africa, Latin-America and Asia. In September 1997 the four Flemish Departments of Family Medicine met with the 8 South-African Departments in Durban. The meeting resulted in the "Durban Declaration" defining a strategy at the level of undergraduate curriculum and postgraduate vocational training in family medicine. The 8 South-African departments developed one Family Medicine Education Consortium (FaMEC). This was the start of a journey of 20 years of development of family medicine/primary health care in Africa leading to the Primafamed-network, based on South-South co-operation, actually contributing to capacity building in family medicine and primary health care in over 20 African countries[28] (see Chapter 10).

In 2005 the World Health Organisation started with a "Commission on Social Determinants of Health". Already in 1984 Michael Marmot et al. studied "inequalities in death".[29] Important research in the United Kingdom like the "Whitehall II"-study[30] and in the Netherlands[31] further documented health inequalities in different populations. In 2008 the report "Closing the Gap in a Generation: Health Equity through Action on the Social Determinants of Health" concluded that "Healthcare systems have better health outcomes when built on Primary Health Care (PHC) – that is both the PHC-model that emphasises locally appropriate action across the range of social determinants, where prevention and promotion are in balance with investment in curative interventions, and an emphasis on the primary level of care with adequate referral to higher levels of care."[32]

2008 was also the year of another important landmark in the development of Family Medicine and Primary Health Care: the World Health Report: "Primary Health Care: Now More Than Ever!".[33] I was involved in the peer review process of this report, and the reviewers were all very enthusiastic about the way important concepts like universal coverage, person-centred care, public-health policies, and leadership and effective governance, were integrated and all converged in the interprofessional primary health care team, working in the community. This report was a starting point for a reflection on the role of vertical disease-oriented programs and the need to integrate those programs in a comprehensive primary health care approach. The approach advocated in the World Health Report 2008, was synergetic with the analysis that was made by WONCA, European Forum for Primary Care, Global Health through Education Training and Service, The Network: Towards Unity for Health, when setting up the "15by2015 Campaign", calling for major international donors to assign, by 2015, 15% of their vertical (disease-oriented) budgets to strengthening horizontal primary health care systems, so that all diseases can be prevented and treated in a systematic way.[6]

Moreover, the integrated approach which was proposed in the World Health Report 2008, was a very appropriate answer to the challenge of "multi-morbidity", which became more and more apparent in the daily practice of family physicians: multi-morbidity became the rule, rather than the exception.[34] The World Health Organisation currently supports the evolution towards integrated care in Europe through the "European Framework for Action on Integrated Health Services Delivery" looking at four components: people, services, system and change. At the global level, the World Health Organisation participates in the Primary Health Care Performance Initiative (PHCPI), supporting countries to strengthen the monitoring, tracking and sharing of key performance indicators for primary health care.

In 2013, WONCA President, Professor M. Kidd, published "The Contribution of Family Medicine to Improving Health Systems".[35] The World Organisation of Family Doctors clearly documented the shift of the discipline from providing reactive care for individuals, towards family medicine as an essential component of comprehensive primary health care, contributing to the improvement of health systems worldwide. The recent years saw an increasing appeal on and attention for family medicine and primary health care in various publications. The report of the High-Level Commission on Health Employment and Economic Growth, "Working for Health and Growth: Investing in the Health Workforce", clearly states that "health systems organised around clinical specialties in hospitals will need to shift towards prevention and primary care. Service models concentrated on hospital care should reform and focus on prevention and on the efficient provision of high-quality, affordable, integrated, community-based, people-centred primary and ambulatory care, paying special attention to underserved areas".[36] In its review "Caring for Quality in Health" the OECD (Organisation for Economic Co-operation and Development) formulated as "lesson 1" for the systemic change for optimising both quality and efficiency: "High-Performing Health Care Systems offer primary care as a service that provides comprehensive care to patients with complex needs".[37]

All these developments require an appropriate definition of primary care. In 2014 the Expert Panel on Effective Ways of Investing in Health that I have chaired since 2013, formulated the following core definition in its report "Definition of a frame of reference in relation to primary care with a special emphasis on financing systems and referral systems": *"Primary Care is the provision of universally accessible, integrated person-centred, comprehensive health and community services provided by a team of professionals accountable for addressing a large majority of personal health needs. These services are delivered in a sustained partnership with patients and informal caregivers, in the context of family and community, and play a central role in the overall co-ordination and continuity of people's care. The professionals active in primary care teams include, among others, dentists, dieticians, general practitioners/family physicians, midwifes, nurses, occupational therapists, optometrists, pharmacists, physiotherapists, psychologists and social workers".*[38]

Family Medicine and Primary Care

Conclusion

Family medicine and primary care developed a lot during the last seven decades. It started with the individual care by a family physician, mostly in single-handed practice. The increasing specialisation led to an erosion of the discipline of family medicine in many countries. In the sixties and the seventies there was a growing interest in psycho-social problems, and a focus on improving doctor-patient communication in order to address the bio-psycho-social dimensions of patient care. The visionary approach formulated in the Alma-Ata Declaration on Primary Health Care (1978) challenged family physicians in order to find out where their place in this broader PHC-approach could be. The development of Evidence-Based Medicine in the nineties, with a strong focus on "medical evidence", created an opportunity for family medicine to scientifically underpin its approach to health problems. The attention for Social Determinants of Health was very helpful in broadening the scope of the approach of family medicine, addressing the social determinants of health and rediscovering the message of Alma-Ata. Finally, the World Health Report 2008, integrated the person-centred care with a "health system" perspective, including universal health coverage, intersectoral action for health and appropriate human resources as building blocks for performant health systems. Increasingly, expectations towards primary health care are echoed in policy papers, which challenge family medicine and primary health care to adapt practice, organisational models and financing mechanisms to address important challenges at the crossroads of societal change.

Reflection by Iona Heath

This chapter tells the story of a remarkable career in primary care that spans 40 years and is by no means over. I first met Jan De Maeseneer in about 1980, when we were placed next to each other at a dinner at the Royal College of General Practitioners in London. Almost immediately we realised how much we had in common: we belonged to the same post-war baby boomer generation, we were immersed in our early years as generalist primary care physicians and we both had young children. We were developing a profound and lifelong commitment to primary care as a force for good in the world and as a bastion against the predations of socioeconomic inequality.

Jan took this commitment to justice and inclusiveness in healthcare and applied it first in his own consultations, then in the creation of the phenomenon that is the Botermarkt Community Health Centre, and, from there, in becoming the Head of the Department of Family Medicine and Primary Health Care at Ghent University. From this strong local base in his home city, Jan has supported the development of generalist primary care, focused on each patient's own particular context, values and aspirations, within regional, national, European and global organisations. He has acted locally and thought globally but he has also acted globally. He has been particularly committed to the development of primary care in sub-Saharan Africa, responding to his experience of working in Rwanda as a very young doctor. Rather than embarking on the traditional didactic aid-based North-South programmes, Jan has always been more interested in building and supporting South-South partnerships between different African institutions, with the intention of fostering solidarity and peer support.

Health services with strong primary care provision produce better outcomes at lower cost and with less health inequality. Building on this knowledge, Jan made a major contribution to the groundbreaking WHO document 'Primary Health Care: Now More Than Ever'. This was adopted by the World Health Assembly in 2008 and has reinvigorated support for primary care around the world. Yet we both remain acutely aware of the constant need to defend a broad and inclusive vision of primary care: one that can fulfil its potential to make the world a better place.

Iona Heath, CBE, FRCGP, worked as an inner city general practitioner in Kentish Town (London) from 1975 until 2010. She is a Past President of the UK Royal College of General Practitioners. She has written regularly for the British Medical Journal and has contributed essays to many other medical journals across the world.

Chapter 2:
Dealing with Social Determinants and Diversity

"Doctor, you should come immediately for a severely ill child!" At the indicated address, in a room in the basement of a building with 3 apartments, I find a lady desperately looking at me and holding a two-and-a-half-year-old child that is clearly unconscious. The child does not react when I call his name. The mother tells: "Yesterday Rocky had a fever. Overnight the situation worsened. At first he was vomiting, but then his reactions became increasingly poorer". Rocky never had serious health problems. A quick control of the vital signs: unconscious, heart rate and respiratory rate very high, low blood pressure. I also noticed a generalised rash. Undoubtedly, this child was severely ill. I called an ambulance and contacted the hospital in order to prepare for intensive care. When the ambulance arrived, the paramedics provided oxygen and an intravenous line and transferred Rocky to the hospital. I started exploring the context of the child to find any explanation for Rocky's condition. Rocky's mother told me that she was currently ill, and that Rocky's father disappeared a year ago. It was difficult for her to take care of Rocky, as she was illiterate. She lacked knowledge about how to reach preventive medical and social services. When I visited the paediatric intensive care 2 days later, I was happy to see that Rocky was recovering from severe complicated meningitis. The paediatricians discovered that Rocky did not recognise "the taste of water" as he mainly was drinking cola and eating chips at home. We were concerned about appropriate home care, and with the hospital staff we decided to prolong the stay. The nurse and the social worker of the Community Health Centre visited Rocky's mother intensively in order to assess the possibilities to create the appropriate conditions for Rocky to return home. However, as so many barriers were encountered the difficult decision was taken to look for a foster home to raise the child but with maximal involvement of the mother. She participated in all major decisions regarding Rocky's schooling, health and welfare. The social worker of the Community Health Centre took the role of case manager co-ordinating the different steps in the care for Rocky. The physical condition of the mother worsened and she died when Rocky was 12 years old. Rocky was doing very well at school and was able to find a job in the business of the foster family. At the age of 21, Rocky invited the social worker and me to be present at his wedding ceremony, and later 3 children were born. Although Rocky's start in life was not all that promising, thanks to co-operation between the different actors, the social determinants of Rocky's life were changed in a way that he could develop his capabilities and build a future.

The "Discovery" of Social Determinants of Health in the 19th and 20th Century

"Every year, more than 2 million women worldwide are diagnosed with breast or cervical cancer, yet where a woman lives, her socio-economic status, and agency largely determines whether she will develop one of these cancers and will ultimately survive".[39] The morning I started writing this chapter, this was the highlight at the cover of *The Lancet* of 25 February 2017. It illustrates the importance socio-economic status and availability of care still have for the outcomes of diseases worldwide. This insight is not "new": in 1845 Friedrich Engels described in his book "Condition of the Working Class in England" the living conditions of working people in cities like Edinburgh. "... the houses of the working people in cities are often so close together that persons may step from the window of one house to that of the house opposite – so high, piled story after story, that the light can scarcely penetrate to the court beneath. In this part of the town there are neither sewers nor any private conveniences whatever belonging to the dwellings; and hence the excrementitious and other refuse of at least 50,000 persons is, during the night, thrown into the gutters, causing (in spite of the scavengers' daily labours) an amount of solid filth and foetid exhalation disgusting to both sight and smell, as well as exceedingly prejudicial to health. Can it be wondered that, in such localities, health, morals, and common decency should be at once neglected? No, all who know the private condition of the inhabitants will bear testimony to the immense amount of their disease, misery, and demoralisation. Society in these quarters has sunk to a state indescribably vile and wretched... The dwellings of the poorer classes are generally very filthy, apparently never subjected to any cleaning process whatsoever, consisting, in most cases, of a single room, ill-ventilated and yet cold, owing to broken, ill-fitting windows, sometimes damp and partially underground, and always scantily furnished and altogether comfortless, heaps of straw often serving for beds, in which a whole family – male and female, young and old, are huddled together in revolting confusion. The supplies of water are obtained only from the public pumps, and the trouble of procuring it of course favours the accumulation of all kinds of abominations."[40] It is remarkable that in the description of this book on the living conditions of the working class, the word "health" appears 61 times, mostly in the context of bad health.

In 1842 a civil servant, Edwin Chadwick, published "The Report from the Poor Law Commissioners on an Inquiry into the Sanitary Conditions of the Laboring Population of Great Britain", describing in detail the wretched social and environmental conditions in London, Birmingham, Glasgow, Leeds, Manchester...[41]

Not only social scientists documented the importance of social determinants of health, also medical doctors like Rudolf Virchow in the 19th century were convinced that social inequality was a root cause of ill-health. He concluded that "Medicine is a social science, and politics is nothing else but medicine at a larger scale". Virchow discovered that not only individual patients but also whole populations can be sick and political action "diagnosing and treating the ills of society" may be needed to cure them.[42]

In the second half of the 20th century important population studies in the United Kingdom documented the impact of social determinants of health. One of the largest studies done were the Whitehall studies, observing the health of civil servants over time. They were able to show a strong association between civil servants' employment level and mortality rates from a range of causes, illustrating the evidence for the impact of social determinants of health.[43]

In 1971 Julian Tudor Hart, an engaged GP working in the small mining village of Glyncorrwg in South Wales, UK, described in "The Inverse Care Law"[44] important mechanisms that contribute to social inequalities in health. On the one hand, poorer populations experience higher levels of morbidity and mortality, while on the other hand they receive very often care of lower quality. The paper also documented that the solution was not in market-based approaches that have difficulty reaching whole populations, leading to continuing inequalities. Moreover, Julian Tudor Hart warned for the "simple solution" to find more money for health care through "out-of-pocket" payments, as this can lead to catastrophic health expenditures, especially for the poor. Finally, the paper also addressed the issue of recruitment of health professionals, where the importance of having a "social mix" was emphasised.

Social Determinants of Health at the Department of Family Medicine and Primary Health Care

It was Professor Vuylsteek who, already in his courses in the seventies, drew the attention of the students at Ghent University to the social determinants of health.

In the period 2000-2005 the Department of Family Medicine and Primary Health Care engaged in research on the "socio-economic gradient in health" in the framework of the PhD-project of Sara Willems.[45] Her work focused on the importance of household-level and neighbourhood-level social status and ill health, the inequity in medical care use in Belgium and the limiting and enabling factors in the use of medical care, starting from the perspective of people living in poverty. Also the different attitudes of family physicians' perception of poverty and of poor patients were explored, documenting the difference between a contextual approach of the patient versus a rather "blaming the victim" attitude.

In the same period the World Health Organisation launched the "Commission on Social Determinants of Health" under the leadership of Michael Marmot. I had the opportunity to participate in the Knowledge Network on Health Systems on behalf of WONCA. So, I found myself sitting in the first meeting of this Knowledge Network in 2006 in Johannesburg (South-Africa). Most of the participants were experts in Health Systems Development, health economics, macro-financing mechanisms,... There were only two "family physicians" in the room. We tried to make a point for the importance of strong primary care, utilising the evidence provided by Barbara Starfield (Johns Hopkins, Baltimore, USA) that the strength of the relationship between income inequality and health is reduced by strong primary care systems.[46] At the end of the meeting the participants had to propose topics for review papers dealing with the relationship between health systems and social inequities in health. I proposed a working group on primary care, but nobody showed up – this was not the only moment in my life that I experienced the loneliness of fighting for primary care. Nevertheless, the outline of my poster presentation was accepted and a paper on "Primary Health Care as a strategy for achieving equitable care" was commissioned by the Health Systems Knowledge Network.[47] A team of our Department did the research and concluded in 2007 that primary health care is a strategy to achieve equitable care, provided that the following policy measures are taken:

1. to guarantee universal access to primary health care through an adequate health system (social security system, national health system,...);
2. to make a shift from "vertical disease-oriented programs" towards a "horizontal community-oriented" approach;
3. education, recruitment and retention of adequate staff, improving the clinical and population performance of the primary health care system;
4. establishment of a performant primary health care service, integrated in the district health system;
5. organisation of health systems in an intersectoral network, with crosslinks to environment, economy, work and education at the different institutional levels, and with use of a bottom-up approach (intersectoral action for health), involving civil society.

Figure 1 shows the paper's hypothesis about how primary health care can be a strategy for promoting health equity and intersectoral action. A first prerequisite is a high level of accessibility of the primary health care team: this means – amongst others – no financial, geographical, psychosocial, cultural,... barriers to access. It is essential that the accountability of the team is clearly defined through a patient list system. In her article "The strength of primary care systems" Haggerty notes: "A mountain of evidence shows that low socio-economic status is one of the highest risk factors in those presenting to primary care. It is therefore possible that health systems that support and value high quality clinician-patient relationships might give patients – most of whom are in a lower social class than their clinicians – an experience of respect, validation, and empowerment that translates into lower health inequality".[48] That may explain the finding that countries with a more formal affiliation between practitioners and their patients, in which a higher proportion of patients were highly satisfied with interpersonal dimensions of care, had more equality of self-rated health.[49]

Another prerequisite is that the team should deliver high quality care. Moreover, the team should interact with different networks (education, work, economy, housing,...). Apart from approaching individuals and families, the primary health care team should also address a community, utilising the "Community-Oriented Primary Care" strategy (COPC).[50] The COPC-strategy enables both responsiveness of the primary health care team to the needs and demands of the populations and intersectoral networking, in partnership with Civil Society Organisations (CSO). Involving the community empowers people at the physical, psychological, social and cultural level and decreases the vulnerability to factors that may contribute to health inequity. Moreover, as this COPC-action will address the living conditions of the local population, the exposure of the people to factors that may be a threat to their health will diminish and the differential vulnerability will decrease. Finally, a better education, better working conditions and decreased unemployment, better housing conditions, access to safe food and water, will improve the structural determinants that influence the social stratification and address the "causes of the causes".

Primary health care as a strategy for promoting health equity and intersectoral action

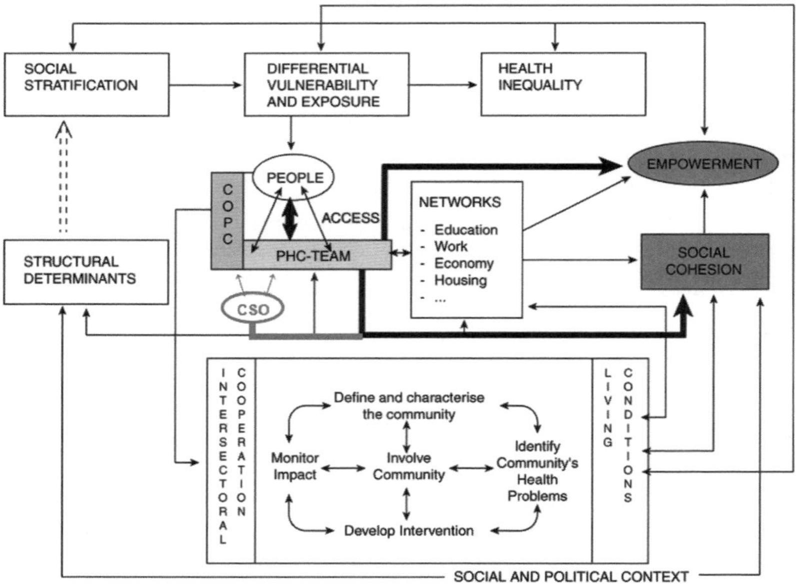

Figure 1: Primary health care as a strategy for promoting health equity and intersectoral action

Family Medicine and Primary Care

Community-Oriented Primary Care:
Health Care for the 21st Century?

Community-Oriented Primary Care merges at the local level, the approach of primary health care with public health. Forerunners in this approach have been family physicians like William Pickles, who in 1931 started to systematically record the name, date, village and diagnosis of all the people with infectious conditions he encountered in his practice. He studied the mortality by reviewing parish records for clusters of deaths. His "COPC-team" was composed of epidemiologists, geologists, a photographer, school mistresses, professional partners, and above: patients. William Pickles over time gathered a community history, performed several specific community diagnoses and, with the co-operation of the community, he was able to intervene with them and on their behalf. By doing so, he improved health in Wensleydale.[51]

Later on, in the 1940s, Sidney and Emily Kark and their colleagues at Pholela Health Centre in South-Africa were the first to systematically implement COPC in their practice.[52] "Actually, Community-Oriented Primary Care is defined as the systematic assessment of health care needs in a practice population, identification of community health problems, implementation of systematic interventions involving target population (e.g. modification of practice procedures, improvement of living conditions) and monitoring the effect of changes to ensure that health services are improved and congruent with community needs. Community-Oriented Primary Care teams design specific interventions to address priority health problems. The team, consisting of primary care workers and community members, assesses resources and develops strategic plans to deal with problems that have been identified. Community-Oriented Primary Care integrates individual and population-based care, blending clinical skills of practitioners with epidemiology, preventive medicine, and health promotion, minimising the separation between public health and individual health care".[50]

In the Community Health Centre Botermarkt in Ledeberg (Belgium) we applied the COPC-approach. Very often observations in the daily consultation were the starting point. For example in the eighties we observed problematic physical development of the local youngsters. This observation was explored through a comparative study on their physical activity, comparing them with the average in Flanders. A considerable gap was shown between the youngsters in the community, who had very limited physical activity, and the average Flemish youngster. In an analysis involving all stakeholders in the community, the lack of green spaces and playgrounds was revealed to be one of the influencing factors. So, not a clinical intervention but the provision of green spaces and the construction of playgrounds were the answer to the observed challenge. Another example twenty years later: when examining the children's throat and mouth, family physicians and nurses often observed the disastrous state of the children's teeth. A cross-sectional study indicated that 18.5% of children was diagnosed with early childhood caries.[53] Children whose parents had a lower education, lower rank in jobs, lower incomes, and were living in more deprived neighbourhoods had a significantly higher risk of early childhood caries. Children whose mother had an East European nationality at birth, had even higher prevalence rates. In a multi-variate analysis the combined impact of neighbourhood deprivation and ethnicity seemed so important that it masked the effect of the other social determinants. This study was one of the decisive arguments to integrate accessible dental care in the Community Health Centre Botermarkt in 2006. In the first year, over 1200 people received dental care. For many of them this was the first time in their life.

Analysing practice data helps primary care teams to address social determinants of health. In terms of priority setting finding the "low hanging fruit" is important when immediate action can make a considerable difference. One of the most useful statistics, which are also relatively easy to retrieve, is the average number of encounters per patient per year in the primary care practice. Analysing the background of patients who for three consecutive years belong to the group of the 10% "most frequent attenders" might reveal important social determinants of health in the community: low education level, unemployment, single, low quality of life,... On the one hand, this analysis may lead to a differentiated approach, e.g. referral to psycho-social care providers, on the other hand this group is informative about the problems experienced by those most in need in the community.[54]

Recently, this approach in which clinical (primary) care is integrated with addressing the upstream causes of ill health (e.g. social and environmental determinants) has been "reinvented" by Merrill Singer and Emily Mendenhall, and renamed to "syndemics", a theoretical perspective to understand the synergistic interaction of coexisting diseases and biological and environmental factors that worsen the complex outcomes of those diseases in population.[55] In a *Lancet Series* on "syndemics" in March 2017 Mendenhall explains how syndemics contrasts with conventional approaches to public health and health care delivery, and explores how "it" can be used to tackle health inequities. Obviously, they never heard about Community-Oriented Primary Care, nor about the eco-bio-psycho-social approach in family medicine. "Syndemics" look like "old wine in new bags".

Dealing with Diversity in Practice

In the last two decades in Belgium the diversity in primary care practices has seen an important increase. Globalisation and migration have led to increasingly changing populations and utterly changing healthcare needs.[56] In 1978, when we started with the practice in Ledeberg, the majority of the patients had a Belgian background, with the exception of a few North African and Turkish families. Nowadays, globalisation has led to a superdiverse community of Ledeberg, counting 106 nationalities on one square kilometre, 95 of them being represented in the patient list of the Community Health Centre. This change has challenged not only the adaptive capacity of communities but also the diversity competences of primary health care providers. Of course, there is the language issue. The community health centre makes use of a wide variety of translation options: "live" professional translators, telephone translation for these languages that are not available as "live translators", video translation, and this in a shared network with local hospitals and other primary care agencies.

However, the most challenging dimension is to understand the meaning of health and illness for patients, the specific epidemiology of certain subgroups (tropical diseases, post-traumatic stress disorder in refugees,...) and the way families and informal networks are functioning. Cultural systems, within and across groups, within individuals and families, have a major influence on people's health and health behaviours. Recently, the Lancet Commission on Culture and Health has brought together healthcare providers, anthropologists and social scientists to extensively review the role of culture in health.[57] Besides the importance of cultural competence of healthcare providers and systems, they draw attention towards social inequalities intertwining with cultural diversity.

In the eighties care providers tried to keep up with the migration streams, studying Turkish culture, culture of people coming from Somalia,... Nowadays this ethno-specific approach is no longer an option and the aim is to function as "ethno-sensitive" as possible. The arrival of refugees from Syria, Africa, Iraq,... introduced the consequences of violence and "human trafficking" in our daily practice. Taking care of undocumented migrants has become a regular task of primary care providers. By law, and unlike the majority of other European countries, the Belgian system provides access to healthcare for undocumented migrants.[58]

Working in this diverse context is not only a challenge, but also an enriching inspiration. To be part of "global stories", when listening to a 50-year old man from Nepal who worked as a truck driver in Europe for 2 years, and tells you that tomorrow he will return to Kathmandu to buy a new house for his father because the old house was destroyed by the earthquake in 2014, broadens and deepens your scope of individual and global experiences.

General Practitioners at the Deep End

Working with vulnerable social groups requires a lot of energy and resilience from the care providers. In 2012 Graham Watt published his paper "General Practitioners at the Deep End", referring to the difficult position of people at the deep end of a swimming pool.[59] In this report, one of the "Deep End general practitioners" said: "I thought about this micro-political level of the every-day stories we hear – people say that it is just an anecdote, it is not real evidence, but that is nonsense. This is evidence... What these people tell us is evidence of whether the system is working or not. Whether society is functioning or not functioning". General practitioners at the Deep End will continue to advocate for political action: *"The social causes of illness are just as important as the physical ones. The practitioners of a distressed area are the natural advocates of the people. They well know the factors that paralyse all their efforts. They are not only scientists but also responsible citizens, and if they did not raise their voices, who else should?"* This reaction clearly illustrates the importance of the advocacy role of primary care providers in deprived areas. The report concludes: *"General practitioners at the Deep End cannot solve the Inverse Care Law on their own. There are three other essential ingredients. First, political commitment and lack of professional opposition to measure and optimise accessibility of the health care system, being at its best where it is needed most; second, national support for the scattered frontline; and third, realignment of local resources, services and structures to support primary care hubs and networks."* Finally, the report stresses the united efforts: *"We do not know where it will end, but it is good to be marching together on the right road".*

The importance of supporting providers "at the deep end" is also reflected in the "Quadruple Aim", formulating the fourth goal of a health care system: "improving the work life of health care providers, including clinicians and staff"[60] (see Chapter 7).

From Insights to Policy

The insights of the Commission on Social Determinants of Health, emphasising the key role of primary care in addressing social determinants, were translated in comprehensive intersectoral strategies, e.g. in the Marmot Review: "Fair Society, Healthy Lives".[61]

Two important messages of this review are:

- To reduce the steepness of the social gradient in health, actions must be universal, but with a scale and intensity that is proportionate to the level of disadvantage. The review refers to this approach with the "proportionate universalism".
- Economic growth is not the most important measure of our country's success. The fair distribution of health, well-being and sustainability are important social goals. Tackling social inequalities in health and tackling climate change must go together.

These messages include important warnings. There is no evidence to create a Network of (Primary) Health Care, specifically for the poor: "A service for the poor is very often a poor service". In the city of Ghent strong efforts are undertaken in increasing accessibility (especially financial, psychosocial and geographical accessibility) of services. Research indicated that in this context also homeless people use group practices and Community Health Centres as the entry point for healthcare, and not emergency departments of hospitals.[62]

Wilkinson and Pickett have brought the analysis on social inequalities in health to a higher level, demonstrating with detailed figures how inequality affects trust, community life and violence and how – through the quality of early life – it predisposes people to be more or less affiliative and pathetic or aggressive. The healthiest and happiest societies are linked by this common factor: the degree of equality among their members. They propose a new political outlook, shifting from self-interested consumerism to a friendlier, more sustainable society. Moreover, evidence strongly suggests that narrowing income differences within rich countries will make them more responsive to the needs of poorer countries: more equal countries tend to pay a higher proportion of their national income in foreign aid.[63]

In a recent series in *The Lancet* on "America: Equity and Quality in Health", evidence is provided that the actual widening economic inequality in the USA has been accompanied by increasing disparities in health outcomes. The life expectancy of the wealthiest Americans now exceeds that of the poorest by 10-15 years. The report documents how the health care system, which could reduce income-based disparities in health, instead often exacerbates them. Poor Americans have worse access to care than wealthy Americans, partly because many remain uninsured despite coverage expansions since 2010 due to the Affordable Care Act (Obama Care). The share of health care resources devoted to care of the wealthy has risen.[64] In an accompanying comment,[65] Sanders, former presidential candidate, writes: *"Health care is not a commodity. It is a human right. The goal of a health care system should be to keep people well, not to make stockholders rich. The USA has the most expensive, bureaucratic, wasteful, and ineffective health care system in the world.[66] Medicare-for-all would change that by eliminating private health insurers' profits and overhead costs, and much of the paperwork they inflict on hospitals and doctors, saving hundreds of billions of dollars in medical costs".[67]*

What is the role of primary care in all this? Not only is primary care accessible through its community orientation, it is cost-effective in its use of resources and appropriate referral policy, but there is also a clear link between strong and accessible primary care and increased social cohesion. To be aware that, when you are in trouble, there is a primary care practice where you can go, where empathetic care providers who know you, will take care of you, and that this service is affordable and accessible for you and your family, creates the feeling of "being part of the society". And this social cohesion is what we need most today.[68] Fortunately, the European Commission took a start on this, establishing a "European Pillar of Social Rights",[69] stating that: *"Everyone shall have timely access to good quality preventive and curative health care, and the need for healthcare shall not lead to poverty or financial strain"*.

Reflection by Graham Watt

This chapter begins with a sensational story about a particular patient who survived and prospered despite the direst start to life. Its relevance to public health and primary care has perhaps less to do with the outcome, which was probably exceptional, and more to do with its active ingredients – clinical acumen, a holistic approach, caring what happened, multidisciplinary support, continuity of care, a long-term relationship, trust. These features are the stuff of general practice/family medicine, but it is only when they are applied to all patients that population health is improved and inequalities in health are narrowed.

The monstrous longevity of Julian Tudor Hart's inverse care law, especially in systems with universal coverage (a misleading term, implying needs-based care but usually stopping short at universal access), is partly explained by the failure of public health "experts" to appreciate and general practitioners to advocate how general practice makes a difference, not only via evidence-based medicine but also via unconditional personalised continuity of care provided for everyone.

Of course the root causes of poor health operate early in life and mostly outside the health system. Health care does make a difference at this stage of life, preventing health problems via antenatal care, family planning, immunisation, screening etc., but also has a major and increasing role in later life via the amelioration of health problems and the prevention, postponement or lessening of complications.

The failure of so many experts on the social determinants to acknowledge this contribution of general practice and primary care, as described by Jan De Maeseneer in this chapter, is itself a social determinant of health. In a double irony, while people with "public health" in their job title tend to have little contact with the public, practitioners with daily and cumulative contact with the public tend not to think about public health.

Jan De Maeseneer has shown the way, building on previous examples. The essential contact, coverage and continuity of general practice make it the natural hub of local health systems, but hubs on their own go nowhere and need to be connected to other community services and resources. Practitioners can embrace or block such change. As Sigerist put it, "They are not only scientists but also responsible citizens and if they did not raise their voices, who else should?"

Professor Graham Watt
MD FRCGP FRSE FMedSci
Emeritus Professor, University of Glasgow

Graham Watt trained in public health, epidemiology and general practice, worked with Dr Julian Tudor Hart in South Wales, led the Glasgow University department of general practice for 15 years and from 2009-16 coordinated General Practitioners at the Deep End, an engagement and development project based on general practices serving the 100 most deprived communities in Scotland.

Chapter 3:

Goal-Oriented Care: a Paradigm Shift for Multi-morbidity?

Jennifer is 75 years old. 15 years ago she lost her husband. She has been a patient at the practice for 15 years. During these years she has had a number of health challenges: hip replacement surgery for osteoarthritis, hypertension, diabetes type 2, and COPD (Chronic Obstructive Pulmonary Disease). She lives independently at home, with some help from her youngest daughter, Elisabeth. I visit her regularly and each time she starts by saying: "Doctor, you must help me". Then follows a succession of complaints and feelings. Sometimes they have to do with her heart, another time with the lungs, then the hip,... Each time I suggest – according to the guidelines – all sorts of examinations that do not improve her condition. As her requests become more and more insistent, my feelings of powerlessness, inadequacy and irritation increase. Moreover, I have to cope with guidelines that are sometimes contradictory. For COPD she often needs corticosteroids, which always worsens her diabetes control. The adaptation of the medication for the blood pressure (once too high, once too low) does not meet with her approval, nor does my interest in her HbA$_1$C (testing the adequacy of the diabetes control) and lung function test results.

After so many contacts, Jennifer says: "Doctor, I want to tell you what really matters to me. On Tuesday and Thursday, I want to visit my friends in the neighbourhood and play cards with them. On Saturday, I want to go to the supermarket with my daughter. Foremost, I just want some peace. I don't want to change the therapy anymore, especially not having to do this and to do that". In the conversation that followed, it became clear to me how Jennifer had formulated the goals of her life. I felt challenged to identify how the guidelines could contribute to the achievement of Jennifer's goals. I have visited Jennifer with pleasure ever since. I know what she wants and what I can (merely) contribute to her life.

Introduction

This chapter originates from the James Mackenzie Lecture that I was honoured to give at 19 November 2011 in London, when I became an Honorary Fellow of the Royal College of General Practitioners.[70]

Presentation of Multi-morbidity in an International Context

Those who discuss multi-morbidity very often emphasise the importance of the increase in "Non-Communicable Diseases" (NCDs). In the 18th century diseases were divided into "Communicable" and "Non-Communicable" diseases because this distinction defined the ward where a patient should be hospitalised: either the "communicable ward" with infectious diseases or the "non-communicable ward" with the "other" conditions. Nowadays, this terminology has become less relevant. When we take the example of the patient with HIV/AIDS, whether he will be "communicable" or "non-communicable" to a large extent depends on the "adherence" to the ARV-Therapy (Anti-Retro Viral Therapy). One of the reasons why the "NCD"-label is so frequently used, could be related to the fact that people think (hope?) that "NCDs" can all eventually be tackled by a selective vertical disease-oriented program (as was done with HIV/AIDS, malaria, tuberculosis and other infectious diseases in the eighties and nineties).

The vertical disease-oriented programs for communicable diseases have shown to foster duplication and inefficient use of resources. They produce gaps in the care of patients with multiple comorbidities, and reduce capacity by pulling health care workers out of the general care in the public health sectors to focus on single diseases.[6] Therefore, in 2009 the World Health Assembly's Resolution WHA62.12 urged member states "to encourage that vertical programs, including disease-specific programs, are developed, integrated and implemented in the context of integrated primary health care".[71] In the domain of chronic conditions and multi-morbidity the focused selective solution pursued for infectious diseases must give way to a comprehensive and sustainable primary health care strategy.[72]

The number of people dying as a result of chronic conditions has risen to 36.1 million deaths per year worldwide, which means that almost 2 out of 3 deaths are attributable to chronic conditions:[73] 22.4 million of these deaths arise in the poorest countries, and 13.7 million in high-income and upper-middle-income countries. Chronic conditions don't merely kill older people, 63% of premature deaths in adults (age 15-69 years) are attributable to chronic conditions. As life expectancy has increased in developed countries, chronic conditions have also become more and more prevalent, and this has been accompanied by a rise in multi-morbidity: 50% of the 65+ have at least 3 chronic conditions, whereas 20% of the 65+ have at least 5 chronic conditions.[74] In the case of Chronic Obstructive Pulmonary Disease (COPD) e.g. more than half of the patients have at least one comorbid disease.[75]

In 2012 Karen Barnett et al. published "The Epidemiology of Multi-morbidity", in which she documented that 23.2% of the people were multi-morbid, with an increased prevalence in people aged 65 years and older. An interesting finding was again that the absolute number of people with multi-morbidity was higher in those younger than 65 years. Moreover, compared to the most affluent people, multi-morbidity occurred 10 to 15 years earlier in poorer people with an important contribution of mental health disorders.[76] Several HIV/AIDS studies[77] [78] [79] have also demonstrated an increased incidence of heart disease, diabetes mellitus, kidney disease, liver disease, osteoporosis, and possibly COPD[80] in HIV/AIDS patients compared to age matched HIV-uninfected controls, an observation which clearly creates important challenges for developing countries.

How Do We Address Patients' Chronic Conditions?

In recent years both Western and developing countries have implemented "chronic disease management programs" in order to improve care. The design of those programs includes most frequently: strategies for case-finding;

protocols describing what should be done and by whom; the importance of information and empowerment of the patient; and the definition of process- and outcome-indicators that may contribute to the monitoring of care. Incentives have also been defined in order to stimulate both patients and providers to adhere to guidelines. This development has led to spectacular results e.g. in process- and intermediate, disease-oriented outcome indicators in the United Kingdom under the Quality and Outcomes Framework[81] (see Chapter 9). The "chronic disease management" approach has led to an acceleration of the implementation of the subsidiarity principle in primary health care with important task-shifting from physicians to nurses, dieticians, health educators, and others. These programs have received positive feedback from providers, patients and politicians, with some critical reflections with respect to equity,[82] [83] to the sustainability of the quality improvement, and to comprehensiveness versus reductionism in health care.[84]

Through a systematic review on effective interventions for chronic diseases, E.H. Wagner (Seattle, USA) described in 1998 the components of the Chronic Care Model (CCM).[85] He emphasised the need for changes both at the level of health systems (through health care organisation) and at the community level (through resources and policies) with an emphasis on self-management support, changes at the delivery system design and appropriate decision support in the context of effective clinical information systems. All these changes should foster "productive interactions" (in Europe, we would say "warm, human interactions") between an informed, activated patient and a prepared, pro-active practice team, and lead to improved outcomes. The CCM has inspired policy makers and providers all over the world and is widely accepted in North America, Europe and Australia. A survey of "Chronic Disease Management" in 10 European countries illustrated that in most of the countries disease management programs are organised per chronic condition, sometimes focusing on subgroups within a specific chronic disease. The 5 conditions that were most frequently addressed are: cancer, cardiovascular disease, COPD, depression and diabetes. Most of the programs use a vertical disease-oriented approach. By most accounts they have led to improved systems for identifying, tracking, and managing patients with individual chronic health conditions. But taking into account the epidemiological transition, we are faced with the question: "How will this work in a situation of multi-morbidity?"

The Story of Jennifer
(See Box on Page 57)

According to the actual guidelines, Jennifer is faced with a number of recommended tasks:[86] joint protection, aerobic exercise, muscle strengthening, motion exercising, self-monitoring of blood glucose, avoiding environmental exposure that might exacerbate COPD, wearing appropriate foot wear, limiting intake of alcohol, maintaining body weight. She should be advised to receive patient education regarding diabetes self-management, foot care, osteoarthritis and COPD medication delivery system training. If she followed the guideline-based recommendations, her medication schedule would include 11 different drugs, with a total of 20 administrations a day. Clinical tasks for the family physician would include vaccination, blood pressure control at all clinical visits, evaluation of self-monitoring of blood glucose, foot examination, laboratory tests... Moreover, referrals would be needed to physiotherapy, for ophthalmologic examination and pulmonary rehabilitation. So, Jennifer's reaction does not come unexpectedly.

The Concept of "Goal-Oriented Care"

In 1991 Mold, Blake, and Becker[25] already recognised that a care model focused on eradication of disease and prevention of death is not well suited to the management of chronic illnesses (see Chapter 1). They proposed a goal-oriented approach that encourages each individual to achieve the highest possible level of health as defined by that individual. This represents a more positive approach to health care, characterised by greater emphasis on individual strengths, capabilities and resources. In Goal-Oriented Care clinicians encourage individuals to achieve their maximum health potential while striving toward individually defined goals. The evaluator of success is the patient, not the physician. In a context of multi-morbidity a goal-oriented approach to health care even makes more sense, because when the to-do lists become too long and too complex it makes sense to prioritise. And the most rational way to do that is that the patient first ascertains goals.

The challenge is to find appropriate ways to explore the "life goals" of patients. How can the patient and his/her goals really be at the forefront of clinical care? In a NICE guideline on multi-morbidity only 1 out of 443 pages deals with "establishing patient preferences, values and priorities" as a strategy to care for people with multi-morbidity. Goal-Oriented Care starts with what the patient wants. The question of the physician is no longer "What's the matter with patient X?", but sounds "What matters to patient X?". This approach enhances capabilities rather than repairing inabilities, which stimulates patient self-management and generates resilience against distress.

New Concepts Require New Research Methods

Exploring the effects of Goal-Oriented Care through research will require new types of research and new research designs and methods. In order to better understand the goals of the patients, new research frameworks and research disciplines will be needed. Disciplines that contribute to the understanding of provider-patient interaction such as medical philosophy, sociology and anthropology are essential. Mixed-method research will shift from purely quantitative (Randomised Controlled Trials: RCTs) towards qualitative approaches (focusing on understanding through in-depth interviews, focus groups,...). Researchers have to look for research tools and approaches that focus on subjective determinants of well-being, and not only looking at biomedical parameters. In the new research designs, patients with multi-morbidity will be the rule (instead of an exclusion criterion), and complexity will be embraced instead of avoided. The International Classification of Function (ICF)[87] might become as important as the International Classification of Diseases (ICD), as it defines a conceptual framework in which different domains of human functioning are integrated. These domains are classified from an eco-bio-psycho-social viewpoint by means of a list of body functions and structures, and a list of domains of activity and participation. As an individual's functioning and disability involves a context, the ICF includes a list of environmental factors and the concept of personal factors in its framework. The ICF is part of the "Family of International Classifications" (FIC) and meets the standards for health related classifications as defined by the WHO. Although the ICD has a dominating role in health care data management, the WHO aims to reach the same level with the ICF, a frame of reference and a classification that is able to define functional status, irrespective of the underlying health condition.

Goal-Oriented Care: from Theory to Practice

Even though Goal-Oriented Care is promising when addressing multi-morbidity, the concept still poses many challenges to providers for adapting it in practice. One of them involves the explanation of the concept of Goal-Oriented Care to patients and their families. When it comes to goal identification, patients experience important challenges which may actually reflect the impact of a health system that is still too much focused on diseases instead of people[88] and a cultural and political climate where the voices of "common people" are hardly heard. Nowadays, understanding processes in relation to the disease, self-determination and self-agency are highly valued by patients. For many people, giving meaning to the chronic illness process they are going through, is of utmost importance. Safety and avoiding side effects (not having to suffer more from the treatment than from the disease) matters. The question is how to empower patients, how to let patients identify personal goals and integrate goals into a bio-psycho-social decision-making process. How capabilities rose and responsibilities are distributed or shared between patients, remains to be determined. But goal-oriented health record architecture across settings where patients can have their own input and which helps care providers to take the goals of the patient actively into consideration, could contribute greatly to the relevance and cost-effectiveness of an intervention, especially in multi-morbidity patients.

Multi-morbidity, Goal-Oriented Care and Equity

Conventional frameworks in medicine and public health, such as comorbidity and multi-morbidity, often overlook the effects of social, political, and ecological factors.[89]

When implementing Goal-Oriented Care, there may be a threat to equity, as the way goals are formulated by patients might be determined by e.g. social class. One could wonder how "Goal-Oriented Care" can be reconciled with the "need for prevention", certainly in people with limited health literacy. In some patients survival (prevention) could be neglected in favour of QoL (Qaulity of Life) goals. Moreover, integrating "contextual evidence" implies the risk of taking the context for granted. People living in poverty will generally have lower expectations in terms of quantity and quality of life than well-educated people. So, "Goal-Oriented Care" could contribute to increased social inequities in health. This challenges primary health care providers with how to deal with an "unhealthy" and "inequitable" context. It is obvious that this cannot be a responsibility of primary care providers alone. However, they may have an important role of "signalisation" and advocacy in order to document and draw attention to the problem.

Achievement of individual treatment benefits is in itself not the final argument for promotion of that treatment for all patients. In one of her last editorials, "The Hidden Inequity in Health Care", Barbara Starfield (Johns Hopkins, Baltimore, USA) re-iterates that organ systems based medicine is becoming dysfunctional, because most illnesses nowadays are characterised by multi-morbidity – cutting across diseases and types of diseases and organ systems. Collecting health information disease by disease may mask the greater needs of people who suffer from combinations of different conditions including psychosocial problems. Disease-oriented medicine could consequently become highly inequitable as it cannot address the adequacy of interventions when people have many problems. Diseases are not unique entities; there are greater differences in resource needs within disease categories than across them. We need guidelines that are appropriate to person-focused care, not disease-focused care.[90] Therefore, health systems should be assessed in their capacity to deal with multi-morbidity in an equitable way.[91]

This is where Community-Oriented Primary Care (COPC) comes in. COPC integrates individual and population-based care, blending clinical skills of practitioners with epidemiology, preventive medicine, and health promotion.[50] Starting from observations in daily patient care, COPC makes a systematic assessment of health care needs in practice populations and communities, identifies community health problems, implements systematic interventions, involving a target population (e.g. modification of practice procedures, improvement of living conditions) and monitoring the effect of changes to ensure that health services are improved and congruent with the needs of individual patients and of the community (see Chapters 2 and 7). So, COPC is an essential part of a strategy to re-orientate care towards the needs and the goals of the individual and of the community, and Community Health Workers can contribute to more equity in addressing the needs.[92] It will help to identify the "upstream causes" that lead to social inequities in health.[93] Both communication and education methodologies need to be reviewed in that perspective. A number of ethical issues will have to be discussed in the framework of "Goal-Oriented Care" e.g. in patients with multi-morbidity. This will need alignment at the macro level in the framework of the political debate on "choices in health care" and at the micro level in clinical encounters with patients, when discussing how to achieve the goals they have formulated.

Looking Back at the Future

Looking at the development of care, especially when it comes to multi-morbidity, illustrates the principle that in history we often experience that "circles are closing". In the second half of the 20th century medicine became more and more oriented towards bio-medical approaches, looking for the molecular causes of diseases. The increasing fragmentation of health care delivery, with the creation of specialties, left the family physician, certainly in countries where there was no clear position for the GP in the health system (e.g. no gatekeeping), with a lot of uncertainty. Family physicians were facing a continuous erosion of their task and function. In the seventies the emerging fragmented approach was tempered by a comprehensive bio-psycho-social model, refocusing on the needs and expectations of patients. Family physicians became champions in "the patient centred communication and consultation".[94] However, an increasing focus on psycho-social problems detached the GP from the "hard core" of medicine: caring for "real diseases". In the nineties evidence-based medicine and clinical epidemiology brought family physicians back to the debate on how to diagnose and treat diseases. Family physicians and public health professionals were in the forefront of the development of critical appraisal of results of clinical trials (see chapter 1). GPs started to develop guidelines, but had to rely on the available evidence, that was disease-oriented and did not look at comorbidity, a key feature of family medicine. Clinical trials, conceived in family practice starting from presentations defined by clinical symptoms, helped to illustrate the complexity and opened new ways for research. Paradoxically, the contradictions that arose when implementing disease-specific guidelines for multi-morbidity patients, brought us back to a need for integration at the patient level, the rebirth of person- and people-centred care, looking at the goals of the patient and combining medical and contextual evidence.[27] In order for family physicians to make this happen, there will be a need for a "new professionalism"[95] and "modern medical generalism" that enables them to guide patients through complexity.[96]

At the same time, it is interesting to discover how fundamental research on the "mechanisms of disease" reveals a unity of concepts: there are common pathophysiological mechanisms to different chronic diseases (e.g. genetic concepts, inflammatory reactions of immune-ageing, chronic systemic inflammation). So, on the one hand the "unity of fundamental concepts" and on the other hand the "unity of the integrated approach to the patient" brings us back to an era of integration, comprehensiveness and synthesis. The circles are closing...

Conclusion

Approaching a patient with multi-morbidity challenges both practitioners and researchers. It challenges institutions for health professionals' education to train providers that are not only "experts" or excellent "professionals", but that are "change agents"[97] (see Chapter 7) who continuously improve the health system by questioning the knowledge and care, as did James Mackenzie. It asks for a fundamental reflection on the individual provider-patient interaction, on the need for a paradigm shift from problem-oriented to Goal-Oriented Care and on organisation of the health care services and the features of the health system. Most fundamentally, it will also require dialogue and communication methodologies between the health sector and people in need of health care, and with stakeholders in other sectors within society (labour, welfare, education, housing,...) involved in health care at the practice, research and policy level, in order to guarantee the essential characteristics of an effective health system, able to function at the Crossroads of Societal Change: relevance, equity, quality, cost-effectiveness, sustainability, person- and people-centredness and innovation.

Reflection by James Mold and Zsolt Nagykaldi

The need for a different approach to health and health care has arisen in large part because of the success of the disease-oriented approach to health care and public health. The prevention, control, and management of infectious diseases and injuries has extended life and shifted the epidemiology of health challenges toward chronic conditions resulting from longer term exposures to unhealthy behaviors and environmental hazards. The ability to identify abnormalities in anatomy, physiology, and biochemistry has resulted in an unmanageable and unaffordable number of tests and treatments, and the field of genomics is still in its infancy. As a negative consequence, the disease-oriented approach has resulted in fragmented and, too often, mechanical, even hazardous care.

When the concern of health care professionals and their patients was on acute, life-threatening problems, it was reasonable to assume that identifying and curing disease would accomplish patients' goals (survival free of serious disabilities). Now that health challenges have become more complex and chronic, and diagnostic and management options more sophisticated, that assumption is no longer valid. Particularly when patients have multiple chronic health conditions or even multiple risk factors (i.e., all of us once our genomes have been mapped), prioritisation is necessary, and the only rational way to prioritise is to reinsert the step of *goal setting* that has, to this point, been skipped in medicine.

Goal-oriented or goal-directed health care, an approach that we suggested a quarter century ago, finally appears to be gaining traction. This chapter is but one notable example. Readers interested in learning more about goal-directed care are encouraged to visit www.goaldirectedhealthcare.org, where they will find additional information as well as a list of published articles on the subject.

James W. Mold, M.D., M.P.H.
George Lynn Ross Emeritus Professor of Family and Preventive Medicine
University of Oklahoma Health Sciences Center, OKC, OK, U.S.

Zsolt Nagykaldi, Ph.D.
Associate Professor and Director of Research
University of Oklahoma Health Sciences Center, Department of Family and Preventive Medicine

Chapter 4:

Decision-Making in Care and Prevention: a Complex Task

September 1986. When I arrive in the consultation room at the Community Health Centre, an incoming phone call by patient Luc V. (48 years old) requires my attention: "Doctor, since yesterday evening I have had severe stomach pain. I have not been able to sleep. I know that normally you only start at 9 o'clock, but... can I please come and see you now? I'm rather anxious about what is happening".

I invite Luc to come to the Health Centre and to see me immediately. He tells me that he has a very busy life in the garage he runs. Yesterday he visited a friend in the hospital who underwent heart surgery. He had a quick meal and then visited his brother, who was recently diagnosed with a brain tumour. Returning home in his car, he felt a pain, not easy to describe in his stomach, radiating to the back. Pain came and went away again and finally was continuously present. "My wife told me I was rather pale, and sometimes my left arm felt painful too. The situation improved, but I would appreciate it very much if you would look carefully at this problem".

Listening to the story, I started to construct a "diagnostic landscape": maybe a gastritis or a gastric ulcer? Or a problem with the gall bladder? Or "hyperventilation syndrome" due to stress? Or could it be acute coronary syndrome (acute myocardial infarction) as I had known the patient for peripheral arterial obstructive vascular disease since 2 years and he was a smoker with more than 20 pack-years, and his father died at the age of 62 from a cardiovascular condition?" And as I knew him as somebody who consulted rather rarely and often late, I had to be cautious. The clinical examination revealed mainly normal findings, heart rate, blood pressure, auscultation,... The electrocardiographic examination demonstrated no signs of acute ischemic disorder. Also negative findings for the thorough abdominal clinical examination, that made the gastritis and gall bladder hypothesis less probable. As he told me that the pain was back and increased, I decided to call an ambulance for a transfer to an emergency department for observation in the coronary unit. A few hours later it became clear that he had an acute posterior myocardial infarction.

Public Lecture in the Aula Mayor on 22 November 1989

In 2015 a follow-up report to the landmark study by the Institute of Medicine "To Err Is Human: Building a Safer Health System",[98] the Institute added that "The delivery of health care has proceeded for decades with a blind spot: diagnostic errors – inaccurate or delayed diagnoses – persist throughout all settings of care and continue to harm an unacceptable number of patients".

Family physicians working at the frontline between society and the health system, play an important role in the quality of diagnosis, with the double challenge: on the one hand to make sure that those people with non-life-threatening, often self-limiting conditions, are reassured, whilst those who present serious conditions, receive immediate action and care.

On Wednesday 22 November 1989 I had to give a "public lecture" to fulfil the last requirements in the academic exam in order to become "Aggregated for Higher Education". In the eighties, after the public defence of a PhD thesis, this was the last part of the procedure. "Diagnostic Strategies in Family Medicine" was the title I was given by the jury.

These lectures were a special public festivity, organised in the "Aula Mayor" of the University, with obligatory "dress suit" ("tail-coat"). My intention was to start with a video of a family physician-patient encounter, but this was impossible, as the infrastructure of the historical building did not allow for video projection. So we used a set of slides, with the conversation on an audiotape, to present the interaction (the consultation is summarised in the box on the previous page). This chapter is based on that public lecture.

Diagnostic Strategies in Family Medicine and Primary Care

In their landmark publication *Clinical Epidemiology: a Basic Science for Clinical Medicine*[99] Sacket et al. described four key diagnostic strategies. First is the "Pattern-Recognition Approach": the diagnosis "on the spot". Family physicians very often use this approach e.g. when assessing dermatological problems, neurological symptoms,... The second is the "Multiple-Branching Method", where the physician follows a kind of algorithm. A "pathway" informs the diagnosis step-by-step. Nowadays there are a lot of (computerised) algorithms available e.g. for chest pain. The third strategy is the "Exhaustion Method": in this approach all relevant medical data related to a patient are collected following a standard pattern and then a careful selection of data leads to the diagnosis. This strategy is often used in patients with complex conditions in secondary and tertiary care. Finally, the most used strategy is the "Hypothetico-deductive Strategy": starting from a limited number of data (symptoms, signs) in relation to a patient, a shortlist of possible "working diagnoses" is quickly formulated. Then specific questions, clinical and para-clinical investigations help to reduce the list of "working diagnoses" as soon as possible, leading to the final "diagnosis". The theory of clinical reasoning that underpins this approach whereby "working diagnoses" or "hypotheses" are advanced early in the patient encounter, and then subsequently tested through additional data gathering, originated from studies, dominated by a psychological perspective, in the 1970s and 1980s.[100] Research in 1988 indicated that, implementing this approach, primary care physicians found the correct diagnosis based on just the chief complaint in 78% of the cases.[101]

Family physicians build their "diagnostic landscape" on different types of information: first of all the epidemiological data (the incidence and prevalence of diseases in primary care settings, age- and gender-specific); the "foreknowledge" about the patient (from the Electronic Patient Record or from the provider's memory); encyclopedical information (as presented in the classical text books that document exhaustively all the "differential diagnoses"); factors related to the doctor (e.g. recently "missed diagnoses"); the "history" of the physician with this patient (e.g. the fact whether a patient is consulting quite "rapidly" for minor illnesses or not, whether a patient is rather anxious or not);

recent continuous medical education activities, "case reports" by colleagues, scientific articles,...; "signals" from the patient (when a patient formulates his own "diagnosis" of the problem or provides contextual information e.g. stressful events); the likelihood of a "serious, urgent condition", and the need and opportunities for quick interventions.

Very often, in a first approach, the family physician will only use two diagnoses: "it is Okay" or it is "not Okay", expressing a sense of reassurance or a sense of alarm. In the literature, this has been designated as the "gut feeling" of the family physician.[102] But, there is evidence for this phenomenon: in a project where family doctors had to assess the condition of 315 patients who called them for "chest pain", in 28% of the cases the family physicians had the feeling that it was "not Okay". From those patients where the family physician assessed the situation as "not Okay", 31% had a serious pathology, whilst only 6 out of 228 patients where incorrectly assessed as "Okay".[103]

Diagnostic Reasoning: Two (or Three?) Tracks

Traditionally the literature on diagnostic reasoning (mainly from a psychological perspective) describes "dual process models" of thinking. The thinking involves two systems: the faster system, Type 1, is automatic, unconscious and seemingly effortless, whereas the slower system, Type 2, is controlled, conscious and effortful. Or in other words, Type 1 is "intuitive, heuristic" and Type 2 is "reflective, analytic".[104] Daniel Kahneman, Nobel Prize winner in economic science in 2002, described in his book *Thinking, Fast and Slow* the relevance of the two types of thinking in different domains.[105]

When family physicians are generating "hypotheses" or "working diagnoses", they use the Type 1 system in the framework of the medical problem-solving process. Experienced physicians in routine cases will automatically retrieve the correct diagnostic hypothesis, based on only a few relevant signs and symptoms. As indicated earlier, the "pattern-recognition" strategy is a typical example of this approach. Very often, physicians use recognition of similarity to a previous seen patient, as stored in their memory. In family medicine, contextual factors such as age, gender, prior medical history, social determinants,... play an important role in generating accurate diagnostic hypotheses, since they may make the presence of a disease more likely or less likely. Sometimes, family doctors know the way their patients normally behave or speak very well, enabling them to compare this with the current presentation in a consultation. The Type 2 approach is mostly used in the framework of "medical decision-making", when a physician assesses the likelihood that a certain hypothesis, generated in the framework of the building of a "diagnostic landscape" to be the correct diagnosis, is tested.

In order to do so, medical decision-making makes use of a rule that has been discovered by reverend Thomas Bayes, who formulated a simple, one-line theorem more than 200 years ago: "by updating our initial belief about something with objective new information, we get a new and improved belief". The background of this theorem lays in a religious controversy in England in the 1740s: "Can we make rational conclusions about God based on evidence about the world around us?" Later on, a Frenchman, Pierre Simon Laplace discovered the rule on its own in 1774. Bayes' rule nowadays plays an important role in matters as diverse as cryptography, assurance, the investigation of the connection between smoking and cancer and Alan Turing used it to decode the German Enigma cipher and arguably saved the Allies from losing the Second World War.

To apply Bayes' rule, there is the general equation:

$$P(A\backslash B) = \frac{P(A)P(B\backslash A)}{P(B)}$$

in which A is a hypothesis and B is data.

To illustrate:

$$\begin{pmatrix} Probability\ of \\ cancer\ given \\ a\ positive \\ mammogram \end{pmatrix} = \begin{pmatrix} Probability\ of \\ a\ positive \\ mammogram\ among \\ cancer\ patients \end{pmatrix} \times \begin{pmatrix} \dfrac{Probability\ of\ having}{breast\ cancer} \\ \dfrac{Probability\ of\ a}{positive\ mammogram} \end{pmatrix}$$

Why did this simple mathematical rule come at the centre of statistical debates? The answer is simple: at its heart Bayes runs counter to the deeply held conviction that modern science requires objectivity and precision. Bayes' rule is a measure of belief. And it says that we can learn even from missing and inadequate data, from approximations, and from ignorance.[106] And that is exactly why it is so helpful for family physicians in primary care.

Fortunately, when family physicians implement Bayes' rule, they are not at all aware about the controversy that lasted for 200 years. They simply look at a possible diagnoses from their "diagnostic landscape", then apply a test (a question, a clinical examination, a lab test, an ECG, another test,...), and then they look at the impact of applying this test on a possible diagnosis with a certain "prior probability", e.g. 0.3 or 30%, apply Bayes' rule, and find the "posterior probability". This will tell them whether or not they have to keep this hypothesis in their diagnostic landscape as a possible diagnosis for this patient. But physicians do this approximatively: the prior probabilities are based on their knowledge of patients and their expertise, and is usually expressed from "very unlikely" to "almost certain". Furthermore, the power of a diagnostic test to confirm or exclude is mostly assessed in terms like "insignificant, weak, good, strong or very strong" and finally family physicians use their own estimated decision thresholds, in order to decide if there is enough "certainty" to confirm a diagnosis, or to reject a diagnosis, or that we are still in the area where further investigation and testing is needed.

According to the Dutch family physician Erik Stolper, apart from Type 1-approach (medical problem-solving) and Type 2-approach (medical decision-making), there is a third track in diagnostic reasoning namely "intuition" or "gut feeling", with 2 aspects: "a sense of reassurance" and "a sense of alarm". In his view the prognostic reasoning starts from "signs and symptoms" and "contextual information" and enters in a process that uses a combination of analytical reasoning and non-analytical reasoning in a circular way navigating between "gut feeling", "medical problem-solving" and "medical decision-making", finally leading to the most probable diagnosis.[107] Many family physicians use the phrase: it fits or it does not fit in. They explain this as a process of comparing pictures, that is comparing the current picture which the overall picture they expect based on what they know about a patient or about a disease. In the case of a sense of reassurance, the current picture is compatible with the known pattern for the patient or for the disease. There is congruity.

In the case of a sense of alarm, there is a discrepancy between the pictures. Things do not fit in; something is lacking, or just off, but the family physician does not (or does not yet) know exactly what.[102]

"The sense of alarm" can be seen as a first warning sign that this is probably "not Okay", which sometimes will lead to prompt intervention, bypassing a diagnosis. Looking back at the patient described in the box at the start of this chapter, the diagnostic landscape originated from clinical science ("stomach pain"), hyperventilation syndrome (stressful context with friend and brother), acute coronary syndrome (risk factors: smoking and presence of arterial obstructive vascular disease), and the important contextual information that it was the first time that this patient called for an urgent visit and presented with anxiety out-of-hours. Utilising Bayes' rule, based on the clinical examination stomach problems could be eliminated, there was certainly stress and the "gut feeling" indicated the possibility for acute coronary syndrome (reinforced by the risk factors). A correct interpretation of the absence of acute ischemic disorder signs on the electrocardiographic recording (a weak argument to rule out acute myocardial infarction), led – in the absence of a "final diagnosis" – to the correct decision of referring the patient to a "coronary unit" in the hospital for further observation. The possibility of a "negative expected course/ prognosis" motivated the decision.

Dealing with Uncertainty

Diagnosis in family medicine is a complex task. For many trainees it is a difficult challenge to learn to deal with "uncertainty". When a family physician is on duty, and he is called 20 times for "chest pain", only 1 or 2 of those 20 patients should be referred to the hospital for further investigation. That means that 18 or 19 should be reassured and advised to stay at home. Students, during their training in family medicine, have to make the distinction between clinical and scientific knowledge, which lies in the fact that scientists aim to discover general patterns and laws, whereas clinicians are focused on individual cases and specific relationships between general patterns.[108]

To accept this "diagnostic uncertainty" and to learn to deal with individual, contextual, and temporal dimensions of clinical reasoning is a difficult process.

Medical problem-solving and medical decision-making accompanied by "gut feeling" and a lot of experience, may contribute to finding the "diagnostic trust" that enables the family physician to function. So, they will be able to work with the complex and often uncertain types of knowledge and their mutual relationships in their profession.[109]

Decision-making in Prevention: Preventing Disease or Preventing Harmful Medicine?

If the management of a patient with an acute coronary syndrome can be situated on one side of the broad spectrum of all possible patient-family physicians interactions, then prevention should be placed on the other end, where the patient has no complaints and there's nothing urgent or life-threatening. A person can request certain preventive interventions or family physicians can offer them on their own initiative. This preventive part of a family physician's job is vast, still increasing and very divers. It includes lifestyle counselling, once only vaccinations, management of chronic risk factors like hypertension, hypercholesterolemia and osteoporosis and screening for serious diseases.

At first sight, decision-making in preventive medicine is similar to the decision-making process in patients with complaints: calculations are made based on prior probabilities and relative risk reductions associated with an intervention. But at a closer look it becomes clear that the paradigm of preventive medicine differs radically from "cure and care" with important decision-making, medical and ethical implications. Curative medicine treats and relieves patients with complaints and symptoms, but preventive medicine brings medical interventions into the lives of healthy people. There are no "patients" in primary prevention, only healthy persons.

This implies, among other things, that the probability of developing a disease and the chance to benefit from a preventive intervention are both rather low. If 1,000 women get regular cervical smears during 30 years, only one woman out of these 1,000 will benefit and avoid dying of cervical cancer thanks to the screening.[110] Or, out of 100 patients who take statins for several years in primary prevention because of a high cardiovascular risk profile, only 2 or 3 will benefit.[111] Family physicians and their patients have to deal with a major uncertainty on who will benefit from the preventive intervention. The consequences of preventive decisions can only become clear after several years and only on a population level. The effect will never become visible on a personal level: when a family physician starts prescribing a statin for a patient at risk and 20 years later this patient has been free of heart infarctions and strokes, there is no way of knowing whether this is thanks to the treatment with statins or whether this was the natural course of this patient's life. Neither is there any immediate feedback that the family physician made the "right" preventive choice: there will be no relief of symptoms (because the patient has no symptoms), there will be no confirmation that the patient's life has been saved by the intervention (like the confirmation of a myocardial infarction by a troponin blood test, and the saving treatment of a coronary stent), nor will there be any reassurance that doing nothing was a correct and safe thing to do.

As a result it is inherently impossible for a family physician to build any experience or "gut feeling" in preventive decision-making and this creates a kind of "alienation". There is no real suitable strategy for family physicians to deal with the decision-making challenges in prevention: to blindly follow preventive guidelines ignores the patient's context, personal story and preferences, while offering prevention only on patient's demand risks inappropriate medical consumption, will serve only the worried well, and will increase inequities in health.

A substantial part of a family physician's preventive workload is the management of risk factors of future health problems, like the management of hypertension, type 2 diabetes and osteoporosis. Although this is mainly a preventive task, these risk factors are described and treated as "diseases", and the success of the "treatment" is measured by surrogate outcomes like blood pressure and blood glucose levels. This attempt to apply a "curative" method to a preventive health issue, might perhaps partly remove the decision-making alienation, but along the process the patient risks to be reduced to a set of parameters and laboratory tests. In older patients the combination of risk factors and surrogate health outcomes often lead to a complex situation of multi-morbidity with polypharmacy and intensive and time consuming follow-up protocols, risk of medication interactions and side effects (see Chapter 3). The prevention of future health problems may actually turn healthy citizens into patients.

Screening for serious conditions like cancer is another controversial form of prevention, because the intrinsic mechanism of screening implies that in the pursuit of health, people who feel healthy and have no symptoms have to be labelled sick and treated. This intrusion is justified by the ultimate health objective of avoiding cancer deaths and mutilating cancer treatments, but the evidence that this actually works is often scarce or of mediocre quality,[112] and the side effects are numerous and sometimes deleterious.

The most harmful side effect of screening is "overdiagnosis", through which a healthy person is, as a result of the screening, diagnosed with cancer and consequently treated as a cancer patient, while without screening the cancer would never have caused symptoms in this person's lifetime.[113]

The family physician nor the patient will ever know whether the prostate cancer, diagnosed after a blood-test for prostate-specific antigen-screening, is a clinically relevant or an overdiagnosed cancer. For the sake of "better safe than sorry" the patient gets the best possible treatment, but in the case of an overdiagnosed cancer, harm has been inflicted on this person.

This paradox poses a major ethical problem for family physicians and the entire medical world. Prevention is performed in healthy persons to avoid disease and premature death in the future, but by doing so it turns healthy citizens into patients with multi-morbidity, at risk for drug interactions and side effects, and – in a worst case scenario – into an overdiagnosed and overtreated cancer patient.

Already in the late 20th century some primary care professionals and organisations, like the Nordic Risk Group (http://nordicriskgroup.net), expressed their concerns about this harmful evolution of medicine because it deprives family medicine of its humanity.[114] In 2007 Barbara Starfield, et al. wrote a sagacious and critical position paper "The concept of prevention, a good idea gone astray?",[115] in which they address the urgent need to rethink the whole concept of prevention with the need for societal responsibility and population orientation, reduction in illness and harmful effects, and the imperative to reduce inequities in health.

But it's only a few years since the message of these early voices has resonated in the public debate of the medical community. Since 2013 there has been an annual international conference on "preventing overdiagnosis" and in 2016 WONCA approved a new special interest group on "quaternary prevention and overmedicalisation". The Belgian family physician Marc Jamoulle is one of the pioneers of the concept of quaternary prevention (P4), what he calls *a new term for an old concept: "first, do not harm"*, reminding us of the "clinical iatrogenesis" concept, formulated by Illich in 1975 (see Chapter 1). P4 might become the most important preventive task of family physicians: "to identify a patient at risk of overmedicalisation, to protect him from new medical invasion, and to suggest to him interventions which are ethically acceptable".[116]

Reflection by Ann Van den Bruel

Diagnosis is arguably one of the core competencies of each clinician; patients visit us with symptoms for which they might want treatment but also to obtain information on what is causing them, what will happen next and whether there are any consequences for them or their family.

In primary care, this is done with little help from diagnostic technology such as blood tests or imaging. In most cases, we rely on clinical features to establish whether a patient is okay or not, and what the best action would be. Traditionally, text books include diagnostic information that is based on secondary care evidence. It's only been a few decades that we have come to realise this does not fit primary care: patients present earlier in the disease process, with other or less advanced abnormalities than what would be considered typical in secondary care. Conducting our own diagnostic research, firmly based in routine primary care, is vital to provide primary care clinicians with the evidence they need.

Such evidence has shown that gut feeling plays an important role in our diagnostic process. It increases the likelihood of serious conditions and has been acknowledged as a valid diagnostic instrument since. I like to think gut feeling is the gift of primary care: being sensitive to our patient's (change in) behaviour and other contextual factors, because we have a long-standing relationship with many of them and have been trained by necessity to rely on non-technological diagnostic information.

Red flags such as gut feeling make a serious condition more likely. But often, we aim to rule out serious conditions, which can be especially challenging because the large majority of our patients suffer from minor illnesses, often self-limiting. Balancing between identifying the cause of a patient's symptoms and the risk of additional tests can be a difficult one. In our low-prevalence setting, overtesting and overdiagnosis is a real possibility leading to harm without benefit. This double challenge, picking up serious conditions in a timely manner while protecting the non-seriously ill, should be at the centre of our discussions with our patients, resulting in true shared decision making.

Ann Van den Bruel, MD PhD, is Associate Professor at the Nuffield Department of Primary Health Care Sciences of the University of Oxford (UK). She is the Director of the NIHR Diagnostic Evidence Cooperative (DEC) Oxford, which aims to facilitate the development and evaluation of clinically relevant new diagnostic tests for primary care. Her main focus has been the diagnosis of serious conditions, especially serious infections in children. In addition to her academic work, she also works as a family physician in Antwerp (Belgium).

Chapter 5:
Towards a Socially Accountable Pharmaceutical Industry?

Performance n°1

On Monday, 19 January 1976 students from the working group MORDICUS (see Chapter 1) perform a piece of street theatre at the campus of Ghent University. The piece is a protest against the increasing influence of the pharmaceutical industry on medical students and their education. Later that week, the association of medical students of Ghent University will open its traditional 'Medical Fair': an exhibition where over 80 pharmaceutical companies gather to inform the students about their products (and flood them with gadgets). For the association, the fair is an important source of revenue, while the companies see it as the ideal starting point for a close relationship with the physicians-to-be. Throughout the academic year, individual companies have already tried to soft-soap the students by sponsoring drinks and sandwiches at 'informative' evenings at the association's clubhouse. The street theatre denounces sponsoring by the industry, exposes the mechanisms by which the pharmaceutical industry imposes its products, criticises the profit-oriented production of medication and their excessive price setting.

When, at the tune of George Baker's *Una Paloma Blanca*, the students sing the lead motive of the performance, the crowd joins in:

"Have you got problems with your mother,
signs of headache or of flu,
take this wonderful white powder
and the sky will turn all blue."

And further:
"We (i.e. the companies) *ask prices for our products*
some may think a little high
but that can never be a problem,
pain will pay for any cure."

Performance n° 2

"Pharmaceutical company Alexion has looked for patients with a convincing story to increase pressure on Belgian government."

On 4 May 2013 the Flemish weekly magazine *Knack* publishes an interview with the parents of Viktor. A few days earlier, they appeared on television to testify about their son's immune disease. In the interview they stated that Viktor's survival depends on the availability of the drug Soliris® (eculizimab), with € 250,000 a year one of the most expensive drugs in the world. Under the conditions in vigour at that moment there is no reimbursement. Afterwards, it comes out that Viktor's father had been contacted by a public relations company proposing the interview. The phone call, however, was an initiative of the pharmaceutical company Alexion, producer of Soliris®, and was set up as a performance to increase pressure on the federal Minister of Health. Viktor's parents were not aware of all that. When asked for an explanation, the PR agency does not see any problem: "Ultimately, the patients and the pharmaceutical company have the same objective: the minister has to make an agreement with Alexion".

The case leads to a fundamental debate on the ethics of pharmaceutical companies that try to broaden the indications for their products beyond scientific evidence.

"The Medicine Man of Tomorrow Is Soft-soaped Today"

In January 1976 MORDICUS distributes over 1,000 copies of their brochure "The Medicine Man of Tomorrow Is Soft-soaped Today: Why We Oppose the Organisation of a Medical Fair". In this document the working group explains why they reject the collusion of pharmaceutical and student organisations. Their first concern is that huge amounts of resources are spent on pharmaceutical marketing and advertising. In the seventies pharmaceutical companies used to spend 15 to 25% of their revenue on publicity. Medical representatives or "reps" – professionals who visit doctors to convince them to prescribe their company's products – account for the greater part of the sales budget. A second concern of MORDICUS is the trustworthiness of promotional campaigns and their negative impact on the prescription behaviour of physicians. And marketing strategies go far beyond just distributing leaflets. The edition of 26 November 1975 of the weekly magazine *Knack* describes how Glaxo (a major pharmaceutical company at the time) frequently rewards family physicians who prescribe the antibiotic Ceporex® (cephalexin) with a colour television, a rather precious device at that time. A third concern is that medication itself has become a commodity, in the context of an economy focusing on the steady increase of production and profits. Return on investment is two to three times higher in the pharmaceutical industry than in other sectors, such as the ailing steel industry. Finally, MORDICUS makes clear that it is no longer acceptable that student organisations collaborate with the industry by organising such a fair. By means of so-called "alternative lessons" and debates the working group provokes heated discussions, not only within the student community, but among professors and faculty staff as well. A year earlier, on 22 January 1975, MORDICUS had set first steps, sending an "open letter" to the Minister of Health, in which they pointed at opportunities to reduce wasting money on pharmaceutical marketing. They specifically emphasised that all the costs involved finally were paid by patient and society. "The Medicine Man of Tomorrow..." became the basis of a roadshow with slides on the malicious effects of runaway pharmaceutical advertising. MORDICUS will show it at numerous occasions, in community halls as well as at meetings of local women's committees.

The Great Refusal

When I started as a family physician in 1978, I had to take a clear position in how I wanted to deal with the different ways – overt or hidden – by which the pharmaceutical industry tried to influence practising physicians. It became clear to me that only the "Great Refusal" (see Chapter 1) could actually work: avoiding any contact with pharmaceutical companies, first of all with their reps. Not attending continuous education meetings sponsored by the industry. Refusing any present or gift by a pharmaceutical company. And finally, looking for objective scientific information to underpin therapeutic decisions. We hung up a poster in the waiting room, stating clearly that we would not receive medical reps, and that it was useless for them to post themselves among the patients. Looking back at a career of 40 years, I think this probably offered me six full months of extra time to spend on patient care. A lot of fellow GPs in Ghent decided to do the same. A logical next step was to look for ways to provide physicians with independent and objective information on drugs.

Independent Information on Drug Prescription

With a few colleagues, Marc De Meyere, a family physician from a Ghent suburb and a future Associate Professor of Family Medicine at Ghent University, created in 1978 *Farmaka*, an independent institution for evidence-based information on medication in family medicine and primary care. Their first initiative was the publication of a state-of-the-art document concerning treatment of the most common problems in family medicine. Another initiative was the training, thanks to a grant by the government, of a group of independent drug reps. Their task was to visit FPs and provide them with independent information, comparing different therapeutic strategies, including non-pharmaceutical alternatives for self-limiting problems, and cost-benefit balances.

Farmaka did not limit itself to the Belgian situation, but established links with similar organisations abroad, such as *La Revue Préscrire*, a French journal that had been publishing independent drug reports since 1981. Five years later, in

1986, they founded the *International Society of Drug Bulletins (ISDB)*, together with other partners and with support of the World Health Organisation's Regional Office for Europe. Drug bulletins had already been introduced in the 1960s, when research had resulted in the development of drugs that would fundamentally change medical practice. It was the time the thalidomide disaster (see Box 3) shocked the world, and forced authorities and the industry to pay much more attention to the side effects of drugs and to the risks of inappropriate promotion and use.

Box 3: the thalidomide disaster.

The thalidomide disaster is one of the darkest episodes in pharmaceutical research history. The drug was marketed as a mild sleeping pill, safe even for pregnant women. However, it caused thousands of babies worldwide to be born with malformed limbs. When the drug was tested, animal tests did not include tests looking at the effects of the drug during pregnancy. The apparently harmless thalidomide was licensed in July 1956 for prescription-free over-the-counter sale in Germany and most European countries. The drug also reduced morning sickness, so it became popular with pregnant women.

By 1960 doctors were concerned about possible side effects. There was an increasing number of births of thalidomide-impaired children in Germany and elsewhere. However, no link with thalidomide was made until 1961. Over 10,000 children were born with thalidomide-related disabilities worldwide.

The thalidomide-disaster led to tougher testing and drug approval procedures in many countries, including the United States and the United Kingdom.[117]

The purpose of ISDB is to encourage independent drug bulletins, to promote international exchange of high-quality information concerning drugs and therapeutics, and to network with organisations involved in rational use of drugs.[118] All these bulletins have an independent editorial team, working within an organisational structure guaranteeing editorial independence.

ISDB is still the only worldwide network of bulletins and journals on drugs and therapeutics that is both financially and intellectually independent of the pharmaceutical industry.

The advent of evidence-based medicine (see Chapter 1 and 6) has had a major influence on the availability of scientific knowledge, relevant to underpin daily practice.

Thanks to meta-analyses (the collective analysis of a considerable number of drug trials), it has become possible to acquire the knowledge necessary to develop protocols and guidelines for a large number of disorders.

In 1998 the Flemish *Interuniversitair Centrum voor Huisartsenopleiding* (ICHO, Interuniversity Centre for Family Medicine Training), together with the seven departments of family medicine in Belgium, started the journal *Minerva* (http://www.minerva-ebm.be/), a journal on evidence-based medicine. Their goal is to provide independent scientific information on medical treatment. *Minerva* screens relevant publications from international literature, and in that way underpins decisions in daily practice. The focus is on problems in populations as they present themselves in primary care.[119]

Filling in Research Gaps in Therapy for Infectious Diseases in Family Medicine

Systematic reviews on frequent problems in family medicine have revealed a lack of relevant research (such as randomised controlled trials, RCTs) on a number of frequent infectious conditions. Therefore, in 1990 the Department of Family Medicine and Primary Health Care decided to engage in a research line on such conditions in primary care. In a RCT Professor Marc De Meyere assessed the impact of penicillin versus placebo on acute sore throat. He concluded that acute sore throat does not require additional diagnostic examinations. Antibiotics are not needed and symptomatic treatment is sufficient, except for patients at risk.[120]

In 2003 Professor Thierry Christiaens found that in women with bacteriologically proven urinary tract infection, nitrofurantoin was significantly more effective than placebo in achieving bacteriological cure and symptomatic relief in just 3 days. This finding was confirmed after 7 days[121] of therapy. Professor An De Sutter performed a pragmatic randomised double-blind controlled trial in family medicine on patients presenting with acute upper respiratory complaints and having a history of purulent rhinorrhoea. Her conclusion was that amoxicillin has a beneficial effect on purulent rhinorrhoea but not on general recovery. The practical implication was that these patients can be safely treated with symptomatic therapy, with the instruction to return if symptoms worsen.[122]

Professor Mieke van Driel (Professor of Family Medicine at Queensland University, Australia) did research on the implementation of evidence in clinical care. Starting from a conceptual framework, three types of evidence were distinguished: medical evidence, contextual evidence and policy evidence (see Chapter 6).[27] In a study on the role of quality circles (a Continuous Medical Education program with small groups of family doctors), she compared a standard dissemination of the guideline on acute sore throat by mail with an additional strategy in a pragmatic cluster-Randomised Control Trial using these quality circles of family physicians. Her conclusion was that such an intervention on quality circles of family physicians integrated in the groups' normal working procedure, did not have a significant effect on the quality of antibiotic prescribing. The study suggested that more attention was needed for the context and structure of primary care practice, and more insight into the process of self-reflective learning in order to find clues to optimise the effectiveness of these interventions.[123] In a study in family practices, patients with acute sore throat were invited to rank different reasons for their visit, and the family physicians received an observational post-visit questionnaire. From this study it became clear that patients with acute sore throat who hope for antibiotics, may in fact want treatment for pain. So, an appropriate exploration of patients' expectations about pain management and offering adequate analgesia can assist physicians in managing sore throats without prescribing antibiotics.[124] In an editorial accompanying the publication of this article in the *Annals of Family Medicine*, John Hickner (University of Chicago, USA) concluded that in the management of acute respiratory infections it could be wise to focus more on symptom relief than on explanations of the differences between viruses and bacteria.[125]

These are all typical examples of research that starts from problems presenting in family medicine and primary care practices, that improve our diagnostic and therapeutic knowledge and contribute to more medical, contextual and policy evidence.

Looking at trials in real primary care settings has attracted increasing interest in the last decade. In fact, the family medicine practice, with Electronic Patient Records, creates an excellent opportunity for randomised controlled trials e.g. to document the impact of two different statins on cardiovascular problems and mortality in patients with e.g. diabetes. The plea for bigger and simpler trials, with data at almost no cost routinely collected in Electronic Patient Records, is an example of how this could be done.[126]

TINSTAAFL

"There is no such thing as a free lunch" (TINSTAAFL): the "free lunch" refers to the once common tradition of saloons in the United States providing a "free" lunch to patrons who had purchased at least one drink. Many foods on offer were high in salt (e.g. ham, cheese, and salted crackers) so those who ate them ended up buying a lot of beer. It indicates an acknowledgment that in reality a person cannot get "something for nothing". In 2016 Collette De Jong et al. studied the association between physicians' receipt of pharmaceutical industry-sponsored meals, which account for roughly 80% of the total number of industry payments, and the rates of prescribing the promoted drug to Medicare beneficiaries.[127] The study analysed 279,669 physicians looking at their prescriptions of drugs and identified physicians who received industry-sponsored meals promoting the most prescribed brand name drug in each class. Physicians who received a single meal promoting the drug of interest, had higher rates of prescribing these drugs. Receipt of additional meals and receipt of meals costing more than 20 dollar were associated with higher relative prescribing rates. The conclusion of the research is that receipt of industry-sponsored meals was associated with an increased rate of prescribing the brand name medication that was being promoted. So "there is no such thing as a free lunch". These recent findings illustrate that probably there is only one way to deal appropriately with the marketing strategies of pharmaceutical companies, that is the "Great Refusal", to disconnect completely from these marketing actions.

Apart from the fact that marketing strategies may affect the independence of doctors, researchers, patient organisations,... another important factor is that they influence the thinking about disease concepts. A typical example is the "medicalisation" (Illich): social processes, where the pharmaceutical companies widen the boundaries of diagnoses to increase their market and sell the idea that the complex social or personal problem is a molecular disease, in order to sell their own molecules in pills to fix it (see Chapter 1). A classic illustration is a description of "disease mongering" by Ray Moynihan: "The Making of a Disease: Female Sexual Dysfunction"[128] published in 2003. In this article the author describes how a cohort of researchers with close ties to drug companies are working with colleagues in the pharmaceutical industry to develop and define a new category of human illness at meetings heavily sponsored by companies racing to develop new drugs. The idea was to build similar markets as the "Viagra"-market, but now for drugs among women. From research it became clear that the subsequent meetings about the topic "female sexual dysfunction", starting with definitions, then looking at prevalence, describing tools for assessing the diagnosis,... were all influenced by people having links with the pharmaceutical company Pfizer. Of course, the side effect of such an approach is that prevalence is overestimated, "normative data" are used for a range of physiological variations,... The impact goes far beyond just marketing a drug, it's about creating a "disease" and medicalising life. Another example of the impact of marketing on concepts is the "depression-serotonin" theory. This theory that depression is the consequence of a "lack of serotonin" originated from the fact that in drug adverts and educational material the message is clear: "depression is caused by too little serotonin, therefore our pill, which raises serotonin levels, will fix it". A patient's guide to an antidepressant reads: "This medication may help to correct the chemical imbalance of serotonin in the brains".

Health Professionals Associations, Research and Industry Funding: the Thin Line

The debate about the relationship between health professionals associations, academic research and industry funding started in the sixties and seventies of the previous century. Certainly, already early in the debate pharmaceutical industry realised that change was needed, so in many countries "deontological codes" were established by the companies. In Belgium, in 1976 the General Association of Pharmaceutical Industry formulated "deontological" rules in the interaction between pharmaceutical industry, academics, doctors, pharmacists, health departments and patient organisations.[129]

Although this code certainly raised awareness about the problem in the behaviour of different stakeholders, the line remains very thin as illustrated in a recent debate in *The Lancet* on 29 April 2017. The start from the debate was the decision by the UK Royal College of Paediatrics and Child Health (RCPCH) to continue accepting funds from manufacturers of Breast Milk Substitutes (BMS). This decision was taken against a motion that passed at the annual general meeting in April 2016, opposing acceptance of funding from companies that marketed products within the scope of the International Code of Marketing of Breast-milk Substitutes.[130] It is interesting to look at the arguments put forward by the leadership of the Royal College on the one hand, and those that supported the motion. Some quotations from the correspondence mainly illustrate that the debate has not changed a lot in the last 5 decades:

- *"Donations from industry will be transparent and acknowledged, but we will not permit the involvement of industry, or linking of a name or logo, to any specific output"* and *"we understand the concern that acceptance of such donations (from industry) might be the thin end of the wedge, leading to inappropriate marketing practices. However, we suggest that dialogue with infant formula manufacturers to find acceptable ways forward is preferable to a stance of total non-engagement that could ultimately harm babies"* (Modi N, President Royal College of Paediatrics and Child Health).[131]

- *"Health care professionals are experienced individuals who obtain information and support from many sources. The assertion that they need to be further protected from industry, above and beyond the rigorous safeguards already in place, demonstrates the lack of confidence in the integrity and professionalism of health care professionals"* (O'Brien D., British Specialist Nutrition Association).[132]
- *"WHO's apparent discrimination against the involvement of industry could be interpreted as a violation of the rights of the infant, since WHO restrictions prevent infants from benefiting from research and development opportunities that are available in other multidisciplinary industry-related areas of collaborative working"*, and *"a core governance standard should be that the actors will come together, treat each other with trust and respect, and develop a dialogue that will lead to collective solutions that will ultimately save children's lives"* (Forsyth S., received grants from governments, charitable organisations and industry; consultancy fees from industry, including companies that produce infant formula. Currently receives fees from DSM Nutritional Products, an international ingredient supplier).[133]
- *"We would like to emphasise that the International Code and World Health Assembly resolutions are intended to protect all children – those who are breastfed and those who are not – by shielding parents from harmful marketing practices and unjustifiable claims by infant formula manufacturers. We urge the RCPCH to change its policy in line with the motion"* (Waterston T et al., International Society for Social Paediatrics and Child Health).[134]
- *"We struggle to educate health professionals about the importance of resisting industry's tempting offers and subtle misrepresentation of the facts, and about the unbiased skilled support that mothers need from them to breastfeed effectively. It is surprising that the UK has one of the lowest breastfeeding rates in the world"* (Savage F., World Alliance for Breast Feeding Action).[135]
- *"For decades, breast-milk substitutes manufacturers have courted health professionals with gifts, meals, and education grants. As Abbott Laboratories (manufacturer of Similac brand infant formula and owner of Ross Laboratories) advised their salespeople in a training manual: never underestimate the importance of nurses. If they are sold and serviced properly, they can be strong allies. A nurse who supports Ross is like an extra salesperson"*[136] and *"The only legitimate way to prevent commercial influence is to refuse commercial funding"* (Parry K.C. et al., Carolina Global Breastfeeding Institute, Chapel Hill, USA).[137]

The debate is ongoing, the arguments are quite "stable". The call for independency involves of course the responsibility for governments and public funders to invest in independent research and information of providers and public.

Evidence Based Medicine and the pharmaceutical industry

One of the major problems with which all critical observers have been confronted during the last 30 years, is the recuperation of the Evidence Based Medicine (EBM) movement (see Chapter 6). EBM was conceptualised to come to a more transparent practice for the good of the patient, with first of all an accent on futile treatments applied in the eighties of the twentieth century. Requiring randomised clinical trials (RCTs) was a major step in evaluating unproven treatments and diagnostic tools. Nowadays there is nearly a monopoly of the drug industry on RCTs. The vast majority are now "sponsored" trials where the industrial sponsor pays for the organisation and has also the ultimate power to choose the primary and secondary outcomes, and in case of negative results, to avoid publication of these negative results. RCTs are the building material of systematic reviews and guidelines, the basis of Evidence Based Practice. In reaction to this lack of transparency the AllTrials movement (www.alltrials.net) is asking for full transparency of all data collected in trials but until now this is not the case. The resuscitation and strengthening of independent research funds is also essential to tackle this recuperation.

It is dramatic to observe the inertia of the Food and Drug Administration (FDA – USA) and the European Medicine Agency (EMA), the biggest watchdogs on drug utilisation, on this topic. In the best of cases this monopoly is regretted but these administrations don't take any measures. Asking for Conflicts of interest of experts is now their mere pretext used to counter the influence of pharmaceutical companies on RCTs.

The Scene is Changing: from "Blockbusters" to "Orphan Drugs"

Looking at the pharmaceutical sector it is obvious that the old recipes will not solve the problems of the future. The cholesterol-lowering medication (statins) that started its career 30 years ago is the most recent example of a "blockbuster", a medication that is actually taken by millions of people in the framework of cardiovascular therapy and risk management. On the other hand there are drugs that treat rare diseases, with a very "limited market". Finally, the pharmacogenomics taught us that treatments become more and more individualised and people with the same conditions sometimes need different medication. How will research and development, distribution, access,... be influenced by this new scene? On the one hand there has been a lot of merging and reduction of the number of big pharmaceutical companies in the last decades, on the other hand new small focused "niche" companies are very actively looking at a small subset of therapeutic strategies. Overall, pharmaceutical industry is doing very well from an economical viewpoint. Five major drug companies made more than $50 billion in profits in 2016 alone.[138] In a contribution to the UN High-Level Panel on Access to Medicines, Mariana Mazzucato (Science Policy Research Unit, University of Sussex, UK) states that *"The current debate about medical innovation is characterised by a poor understanding of, and many myths around, the drivers behind innovation, in particular the respective roles of public and private actors in the innovation process... Our current innovation system drives medical research and development's priority setting in the direction of greatest profit but not of greatest need nor of true medical benefit, and allows pharmaceutical companies to charge high prices that have no relation to the actual cost of developing and manufacturing the medicines. Current economic and regulatory incentives have resulted in a highly financialised pharmaceutical sector that fails to deliver the medical innovation we need, despite major public and private investments and rhetoric of unprecedented medical progress. Over two thirds of new medicines reaching the market do not represent any therapeutic advance for the patients, while many health needs remain unmet. In combination with high medicine prices for the relatively few drugs that are medical breakthroughs, our medical innovation system needs a radical transformation in order to respond to social justice imperatives that should govern health and human rights".*[139] Although public sector investments, through organisations like the

National Institute of Health (NIH) in the USA or the Medical Research Council (MRC) in the UK, contributed fundamentally to advances in the industry, the "narrative" continuous to be that it are the large private companies that are the most important (the biggest "value creators" and "risk takers"), and this has justified their power in determining the prices that are set (to recoup R&D costs, as well as more recent "value based pricing" arguments), as well as the direction of innovations.[140] Vallas et al. report an example from biotechnology: *"A new pharmaceutical that brings in more than $1 billion per year in revenue is a drug marketed by Genzyme. It is a drug for a rare disease that was initially developed by scientists at the National Institutes of Health. The firm set the price for a year's dosage at upward of $350,000. While legislation gives the government the right to sell such government-developed drugs at 'reasonable' prices, policymakers have not exercised this right. The result is an extreme instance where the costs of developing this drug were socialised, while the profits were privatised. Moreover, some of the taxpayers who financed the development of the drug cannot obtain it for their family members because they cannot afford it".*[141] Recently, the mechanism of value-based pricing is put forward, which suggests that the value and therefore price of a medicine can be equated to what it would cost to the health system to not have that medicine. For instance, the $84,000 price for twelve-weeks hepatitis C treatment costing less than $200 to manufacture, is justified because it is "cheaper than a liver transplant", the ultimate treatment for people dying from a chronic hepatitis C infection. This is of course an absurd reasoning, as it decouples the price from the "real development and production cost".

These examples illustrate that we need a new frame of reference to stimulate relevant innovation, leading to accessible medicines, and this requires a new relationship between governments, research institutes, the pharmaceutical industry and the public.

Access to quality medicines at fair prices

The Expert Panel on Effective Ways of Investing in Health (EXPH) devoted a chapter from its opinion "Access to Health Services in the European Union" to the problem of availability of quality medicines at fair prices.[142] On the one hand, the Panel states that access to medicines has improved overtime due to the expiry of patents for "blockbuster" products. For off-patent medicines access issues focus on the importance of generics and biosimilars; in general, strategies to increase the utilisation of generics where competition between different producers is more obviously present, have obtained good results. Of course access is always dependent on coverage with financial protection: how well the health system protects people against out-of-pocket payments for medicines. On the other hand, according to the Panel, debates around access to new medicines have intensified. "Key issues here also concern coverage (who has access, within and across countries?) and prices (are health systems able to pay for new medicines?), and extend to thinking about how best to provide incentives for innovation (do payment mechanisms encourage the development of medicines that address unmet therapeutic needs?) and how to balance incentives against the budget impact of paying for new products. These issues have led many to call for a re-think of funding for research and development, and payment for innovation – a complex challenge that deserves a careful reassessment of existing mechanisms and a thorough exploration of all alternative mechanisms, including mandatory licensing on public health grounds when no price and quantity agreement is reached with innovators, and public-private policy initiatives such as de-linking prices and R&D costs where appropriate".

Countries are increasingly working together in the framework of "horizon scanning" for pharmaceutical products. An example is the "BeNeLuxA Initiative-Collaboration on Pharmaceutical Policy" where Belgium, the Netherlands, Luxemburg and Austria work together in order to look for products in development that may have an important impact, both clinically and at the level of the budget. By doing so, topics for intensified co-operation can be identified.[143]

The "polypills", a solution to all problems?

Recently an interesting debate started on "polypills", fixed dose combinations of different products (e.g. aspirin, statin and ace-inhibitor). There is actually a strong tendency, certainly in the cardiovascular domain, to promote widespread use of "polypills" for cardiovascular disease, both for secondary prevention (in people who already have cardiovascular problems), but also in "high-risk primary prevention, based on formal individual risk assessment" and for primary prevention based on single risk factor measurement, such as age, also known as "mass treatment".[144]

One can wonder if this will not lead to further medicalisation, as age becomes a risk factor (I always thought that age was an indicator of successful outcome?). It is amazing to read with which doses of enthusiasm the authors make a plea for widespread implementation, ask for government reimbursement and more dynamic physician uptake.[145] A look at the affiliation of the authors ("declarations of interest") indicates that a lot of them have been paid for development of combination products, others were heavily involved in trials with these products and/or have received speaker fees from producers. Actually, there are only process evaluations, with intermediate end points (change in risk factors), there is no evidence of impact of the use of polypills on outcome indicators (morbidity and mortality). Another interesting finding is that the country with the highest availability of polypills with marketing approval is India, where 7 different polypills are available. In India huge health inequalities are related to socio-economic status, geography and gender, and are compounded by high out-of-pocket expenditures, with more than three-quarters of the increasing financial burden of health care being met by households. Health care expenditures exacerbate poverty, with about 39 million additional people falling into poverty every year as a result of such expenditures.[146] Will the roll-out of the polypills really make a difference and contribute to more health equity in such a country? A thorough reflection on the ethical, sociological, societal,... impact of the worldwide introduction of the polypills as a priority should be started involving all stakeholders. Especially family physicians, who will be asked to contribute to this roll-out, should participate in this debate. Family physicians probably will have problems with the inflexibility of dosing in these medications, the use of this medication for primary prevention (see Chapter 4), the possibility of side effects (where it will be difficult to identify the ingredient that caused the side effect), and the potential negative impact on health-related behaviour, as the polypills are a substitute for efforts to improve healthy lifestyles.[145]

Family Medicine and Primary Care

What Will This Mean for Family Medicine and Primary Care?

The analysis in this chapter indicates that it is key for family medicine and primary care to participate actively in this debate. Almost every week one can find an article in the press stating that "... family physicians should reduce the prescription of particular drugs, e.g. antidepressants, antibiotics,...". Moreover, in many countries, family physicians are accountable for the percentage of generics they prescribe, in order to reduce costs.

Quality of prescribing is continuously an issue in many countries. The largest part of all prescriptions worldwide are issued at primary care level. Interprofessional initiatives, involving family physicians, nurses, pharmacists,... can contribute to better performance in drug prescription. Rational evidence-based prescribing is the key to making sure that people have access to quality medications at the moment they need it and at a price they can afford, avoiding financial hardship.

But here also recuperation is a major concern the last years: the correct criticism that patients are mostly not involved in research was rapidly seen by the industry as an opportunity to find new partners. Patient organisations are extensively sponsored by the industry, specific testimonies are organised to force reimbursement of extremely expensive drugs (see box at the beginning of this chapter), even protest actions are organised as by the UK Alzheimer league near the Houses of Parliament for the sake of reimbursement of inefficient Alzheimer drugs. Here again primary health care has to take its advocacy role to safeguard the benefit of the whole population.

A socially accountable pharmaceutical industry and the availability of independent information on drugs are essential requirements for better answers to the actual societal challenges.

Reflection by Martin McKee

The pharmaceutical industry has a problem. Back in the 1960s it had good reason to be optimistic. It worked through one body system after another, identifying common diseases, ideally with an onset in middle age and requiring lifelong treatment. They hit one jackpot after another. Yet, like all good things, it had to come to an end. The problem was that they ran out of common diseases needing long-term treatment. There were still plenty of diseases that needed effective treatments. The problem was that the number of potential patients was much smaller. In areas such as cancer, increasingly specific targeting by drugs aimed at individual receptors meant that only a few patients might actually benefit from the new treatment, and even they might only take it for a few months. This would make it much more difficult to return a profit.

One way to address this problem was to introduce the idea of orphan diseases, allowing the duration of patents to be extended, so that the longer stream of protected income would be an incentive to invest in their development. But this was not a solution. Take antibiotics. To be profitable, industry had to sell as much as possible quickly. But if it did, it risked antimicrobial resistance. As a consequence, the industry simply stopped investing in this area. Another strategy was needed. If there were no common diseases left to treat, then why not invent them? After all, the normal process of ageing leads to many signs and symptoms. So why not give them a name and, with it, the need for a treatment? All that is needed is to redefine the boundaries of physiological distributions or lowering the threshold for treatment. Soon, thousands of people find they are suffering from conditions such as Low-T (testosterone) or restless legs syndrome, each requiring long-term treatment. Profitability, if not health, is restored. In this chapter Jan De Maeseneer provides an excellent account of the pressures that these developments place on family doctors, as well as imaginative ways to resist them. As he notes, we on the European Commission's Expert Panel on Effective Ways of Investing in Health have been grappling with the problem of how to encourage innovation in the numerous drugs that are still needed. There are many good ideas around, most involving a change to the existing system, where governments, through their funding of basic research, take the risks, while industry keeps the profits.

Martin McKee is Professor of European Public Health at the London School of Hygiene & Tropical Medicine and immediate past president of the European Public Health Association.

Chapter 6:

The Quality of Care:
and the Care for Quality

It is May 1994 when a fifty-five-year-old man comes to see me for stomach pain. He did not have an easy life, lives alone, is illiterate and jobless. He tells that the pain is already there for some months and that he is losing weight, as he had not much appetite during the last weeks.

The clinical examination made it clear that a gastroscopy in order to assess the stomach pain was needed and I explained the procedure to Jack. Most of the patients are quite anxious for this procedure, as a kind of flexible tube has to be entered through the mouth, finally reaching the stomach for visual inspection.

Two weeks later, Jack is back for a follow-up consultation. In the meantime I had received the results from the specialist. Immediately at the start of the consultation Jack tells me: "Doctor, I know that I have cancer. So tell me what to do." I was quite surprised and asked him: "Tell me, why do you think that you've got cancer?" "Well, doctor, when the specialist, at the end of the procedure, handed over the little part that he had taken out of my stomach to the nurse, so that she could prepare it for further examination, I understood from the way the doctor looked at the nurse that I had cancer." I was amazed, and invited him to tell how he looked at this problem, and what his expectations and goals would be: "What really matters to you, now that you know that you have cancer?" For Jack the essence was to have no pain, to be able to meet with his son who lived in France for more than 20 years, and for the rest, if possible, to die at home. So, the "quality agenda" for Jack and myself was quite clear.

Reflecting on this consultation, I realised how important communication between provider and patient is for the quality of health care, and how we should be aware that we continuously "send information to the patient", be it in words ("digital language"), or in the way we behave, look, speak,... ("analogous language").

Background

This chapter is mainly based on our publication in *The Lancet* in 2003 entitled "The Need for Research in Primary Care".[27]

In 1972 Archie Cochrane concluded that in order to improve quality the clinical sector of the UK National Health Service (NHS) should be based on science, in particularly on the conclusions of Randomised Control Trials (RCTs).[147] The idea was that disseminating the results of the trials would directly impact the care for patients. Forty-five years later Cochrane's approach clearly enhanced the number of published papers, but it has had rather limited effect on clinical practice and policies – even when applying the most sophisticated electronic techniques and decision support tools. One of the reasons could be that the notion of quality of care is quite complex, and that we need to broaden the contemporary ideas about Evidence-Based Medicine and look at the need for medical, contextual and policy evidence. This seems especially relevant for primary care.

Quality of Care and Caring for Quality: a Theoretical Framework

Documenting the quality has become increasingly important and doctors can no longer self-proclaim their work and services to be of "high quality". Even after more than 25 years the Institute of Medicine's (nowadays the "National Academies of Sciences, Engineering and Medicine") definition of quality is widely accepted: "Quality of care is the degree to which health services for individuals and populations increase the likelihood of desired health outcomes and are consistent with current professional knowledge".[148]

Figure 2 shows the complex picture of determinants of quality, starting from the Donabedian triangle of Structure, Process and Outcome,[149] and gives a theoretical framework that enables analysis of quality of care.[150]

Structure consists of three interrelated components: society, the individual, and the health care system. Society presents a so-called epidemiological community, characterised in terms of morbidity, socio-economic status, employment, housing, and other variables; a cultural community (referring to an anthropological frame of reference); and a support community, with formal, informal, and professional networks. At the level of the individual, biopsychological status, knowledge (about the functioning of the body), skills (coping and resilience, self-care), and attitudes (health perceptions and health beliefs) affect clinical care. For the health care system, organisational aspects (accessibility, continuity, sustainability) and characteristics of health care providers (competence, empathy, co-operation) affect quality of care.[151]

Process refers to all interventions and interactions between patients and providers. Process quality largely depends on adequate communication, medical decision-making, and management of care. Guidelines, protocols, and algorithms that underpin processes are increasingly based on scientific evidence. Structure and process are inextricably linked in continuous interaction. Quality of communication between patients and doctors, for instance, will be determined not only by the skills of the doctor but also by patients' characteristics (e.g. health beliefs) and by community characteristics – e.g. importance of integration of cultural-anthropological factors in communication with migrants. Medical decision-making (see Chapter 4) will interact with the patient's expectations and beliefs – e.g. it is difficult to make clear to a patient who has unrealistic faith in medical technology that a CT scan is not needed for diagnosis of acute sinusitis. Both structure and process will lead to the final outcome.

Outcome is decided by how patient and provider perceive health and disease, and this perception has shifted from disease-orientation to goal-orientation, especially in the context of multi-morbidity (see Chapter 3).[25][71] As a result – e.g. for a patient with chronic pulmonary disease – the patient's ability to participate in social life is more important than their change in lung-function test results. This consideration leads to a range of relevant outcome indicators that can be measured, from signs and symptoms, physical functions (e.g. blood pressure, blood glucose, peak flow), quality of life (that is increasingly linked to functional status),[152] patient's satisfaction, and social equity. In Figure 2 we emphasise the complexity of the different components of quality, and the picture is undoubtedly incomplete. Moreover, the figure highlights the fact that a linear mechanistic approach is not appropriate to improve quality. What is really needed is comprehensive circular approaches.

Figure 2 also makes clear that Evidence-Based Medicine must not be overestimated in the quality debate. Its role is restricted to improvement of the scientific rigour of guidelines and protocols. An essential aspect of quality of care is the need to value outcomes (nowadays there is an increasing focus on "value-based care"). Evidence-based medicine then allows analysis of effectiveness and efficiency of pursuing these outcomes.

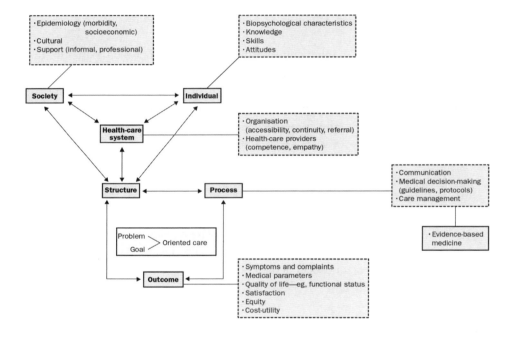

Figure 2. Theoretical Framework of Structure, Process and Outcome
(Courtesy of *The Lancet*[27])

Taking into account the limitations of every country's health care budget, equity (and not cost-containment) is an important outcome variable at the level of society, and implies that three types of evidence are needed: medical, or "professional" because it encompasses nursing, physiotherapeutic, nutritional,... evidence, contextual and policy evidence.

Clinical decisions to improve quality of patients' care must be made with a good knowledge of the disease (medical evidence), but at the same time they must take into account patient-specific aspects of medical care (contextual evidence) and efficiency, equity, and rationing and avoiding waste (policy evidence).[147]

Medical (or better "Professional") Evidence

Although the amount of professional evidence increases daily, many core questions in family medicine and primary care remain unanswered. Clinical questions trigger various methodological approaches, such as decision analysis, meta-analysis, practice guidelines, clinical pathways, patient management, systematic reviews, and critically appraised topics. Evidence-Based Medicine relies – in all these methods in particular – on RCTs that emphasise efficacy: how an intervention works in a well-defined setting for a specific group of patients with a distinct disease. This information is especially for primary care physicians insufficient, because they have to treat less clear-cut illnesses in indistinct patients' groups. In family medicine, tension between clinical research and clinical practice arises because research generally does not include a representative sample of patients with respect to age and ethnic origin or comorbidity, and in the typical presentation of non-specific symptoms of an early disease stage.[153] That is why in primary care clinical decisions are increasingly made in view of symptoms (dysuria,[121] sore throat,[154] purulent rhinorrhoea[122]), and supporting research should also be done with this view, because treatment generally starts when diagnosis is still not known.

Moreover, many patients in primary care have two or more diseases (multi-morbidity), which is the case in elderly people, but also in the group under 65 years there are a lot of persons with multi-morbidity.[76] So, family physicians are confronted with questions like: "What is the evidence to follow in the management of an 82-year-old patient with chronic obstructive pulmonary disease (COPD) and type 2 diabetes, because treatment with corticosteroids could interfere with control of glycaemia? A lot of data exist about treatment of COPD or management of type 2 diabetes for patients younger than 75 years. There is, however, little evidence about how to treat an 82-year-old patient who has both conditions. Probably for the 82-year-old patient it is more appropriate to start with the question: "What does really matter to this patient?", and in a "goal-oriented" approach[70] to assess to what extent interventions based on the existing evidence may contribute to the achievement of the goals of the patient (see Chapter 3). It is also important to realise the relevance of negative study findings that help to identify spurious interventions. This may be illustrated by the effect of studies on antibiotics that lend support to restricted use in case of, for example, acute bronchitis.[155]

Another drawback is that probable conclusions from trials are presented to a physician, who looks for guidance in a definite yes-no decision in a particular patient – more uncertain certainty in Richards' words.[156]

A basic assumption in guideline development is that clinical research follows clinical relevance. In reality, much research is driven by commercial interests.[157] Moreover, the pharmaceutical industry could actively be involved in the so-called "making of a disease", as in the case of female sexual dysfunction (see Chapter 5).[128] As a result, more evidence is published on pharmacological treatments than on the effects of interventions aimed at changing health behaviour. As a result, there is a danger of Evidence-Based Medicine to pursue what is possible and available rather than what is relevant.

Contextual Evidence

Contextual evidence is necessary to assist providers to address the challenge of how to treat a particular patient in a specific situation. This need refers back to the principles of good doctor-patient communication to create trusting interpersonal relationships, exchange of pertinent information, and negotiation of treatment-related decisions.[158] Good communication includes both instrumental and affective behaviours, but there is no blueprint to guarantee a favourable outcome.[159] Factors that affect communication are related to the character and personality of doctor and patient and their personal history (continuity of care), disease characteristics (life-threatening diseases, depression, chronic pain), and family, socio-economic, and cultural circumstances. Conflicts in the Middle East, for example, terrorist attacks,... affect western doctors' communication with patients of a specific ethnic origin.

Family Medicine and Primary Care

The underlying issue is that what comprises a diagnostic method – communication to establish a history or convey a diagnosis – is at the same time an intervention. Here, translation of study findings becomes a difficulty when a randomised controlled trial (RCT) needs rigorous standardisation of history taking, diagnosis, and patients' information. Trial design first excludes part of the regular intervention to assess the effects of the innovative, experimental one, and introduces the danger of overvaluing the new method over the established one. Another drawback relates to selective study dropout: patients from lower socio-economic status – in itself a barrier to use certain diagnostic and therapeutic strategies – might most frequently be lost to follow-up in RCTs. Usually, little information is given about the socio-economic characteristics of patients in the dropout groups,[160] which hampers extrapolation to regular patients' care.

Extrapolation from research to practice presumes that patients are open to a rational approach, take responsibility for their own health, and make their own informed decisions. Evidence-Based Medicine depends in part on these factors, but many patients attribute their health status to external factors beyond their control (external health locus of control).[161] When research offers probabilities and "numbers needed to treat", patients expect certainty from their doctor, wanting to know whether treatment is successful for them. One way or another, physicians have to cope with this expectation, which brings ethical deliberations into the arena. While promoting best evidence care, doctors could be caught in a conflict between their obligation to promote health and respect for the patient's autonomy. To pursue medical benefits over the patient's autonomy can be valued as solidarity with the patient, but also as overprotection and paternalism. Similarly, respect of patients' wishes for self-determination can be viewed as indifference to their medical needs. As the (family) physician has to include these factors in every consultation with a patient, understanding contextual evidence is necessary to bridge the gap between efficacy – what works in isolation in an ideal setting – and effectiveness (what works in routine practice).

Policy Evidence

The health-policy environment decides every meeting of (family) physicians and their patients, and therefore there is a need to enrich practice with more policy evidence, which entails efficiency, equity, rationing and avoiding waste. Achievement of individual evidence-based treatment benefits is in itself not the final word for promotion of that treatment for all patients. An assessment of therapy in Chronic Obstructive Pulmonary Disease stressed this: *"Although the evidence suggests that improved compliance with guideline-recommended practice will improve symptoms and disease-specific quality of life, further work needs to be done to establish the cost-effectiveness of chronic therapies for COPD relative to other chronic conditions. Without such data, payers will be reluctant to allocate scarce resources to expensive guideline implementation programs for individuals with this condition."*[162]

Maynard stressed the implications of resource allocation in more general terms.[163] When there are two treatment options – option A leading to 5 years of good quality-of-life survival, and option B leading to 10 years – an obvious evidence-based choice would favour option B. However, when limited resources are taken into account, and option B is the most expensive option, option A may produce more years of good quality of life than option B at the level of the population. From a population perspective, the evidence-based choice is option A. A clinician prescribing option B uses resources inefficiently, and this practice deprives other patients of care from which they could benefit. Aggregated on a national or international level, individual best quality of care further complicates the division of wealth between rich and poor. Integration of equity and solidarity into decisions enhances understanding of how choices stimulate or impede best practice for all patients. This act enhances transparency of clinical performance, and its importance for the quality culture in medical care. Regulations such as the (non)existence of gatekeeping, reimbursement, and payment, regulations for advertising of medicines, and continuing medical education have an effect on physicians' and patients' behaviour, which goes beyond the limits of the health care system. For instance, in occupational asthma, to change working conditions would be the most logical intervention for the patient. But out of fear of losing their job, patients might prefer symptomatic treatment without notifying the employer of their diagnosis. In such a case, an advocacy approach where the provider supports the patient to ask for healthier working conditions, may be appropriate.

In order to translate "medical/professional evidence", "contextual evidence" and "policy evidence" into practice, the Expert Panel on Effective Ways of Investing in Health identified 5 core dimensions for which goals, standards and indicators should be developed in order to guarantee high-quality health care services:[164]

- effectiveness (improve health outcome);
- safety (prevent avoidable harm related with care);
- appropriateness (comply with current professional knowledge, meet standards);
- person/patient-centredness (consider patients/people as key partners in the process of care);
- efficiency and equity (optimal use of available resources without differences, variations and disparities in the health achievements of individuals and groups).

Translating Theory into Practice

In the last two decades different factors have influenced not only the debate about quality and safety, but also the context in which health care providers have to put this into practice. A first important fact and to some extent probably the most "disruptive innovation" in health care has been the changing position of the patient, who nowadays acts as a "consumer of care" and has gained power. Of course, this is an opportunity, because people themselves can actively contribute to improvement of quality of care. There is an ongoing discussion about the "best strategy": either "intrinsic motivation" or "external control"? Probably both have a role to play, with an active involvement of patients/citizens. Accountability and transparency are key concepts and should be translated in "relevant performance indicators".

The literature on quality improvement interventions is rather disappointing. Many patients do not receive the care they should receive: studies estimate that this applies to 30-45% of the patients, estimated 20-25% of the diagnostic or treatment actions are not really needed or ineffective to improve the patient's health or well-being or even harmful for patients.[165] Just as an illustration: a national audit in 100 representative practices in the Netherlands using a set of rigorously developed clinical indicators, based on evidence-based guidelines, showed that only 62% of the prescribing decisions were in line with national guidelines.[166] Goderis et al. assessed the appropriateness of metabolic control in 2495 diabetes mellitus – type 2 patients registered with 120 volunteer general practitioners. The glycaemic control was achieved in 54% of the patients, systolic blood pressure targets were reached in 50% and LDL levels lower than 100mg/dl were reached in 42%.[167] The list of such studies in many countries that show that actual care is often not meeting criteria for good quality and safety is endless. But, on the positive side, better structured and organised care and interprofessional collaboration give better patient outcomes, motivation in professionals to really work on improvement is key and there is also need for external support in order to reorganise the practice for better care.[168]

Nevertheless, there are some clear recommendations that may help in order to improve quality:

- Evidence and evidence-based guidelines are only the starting point of a process of change. They should be integrated in patient care in a meaningful way. This requires integration of medical/professional, contextual and policy evidence.
- The starting point of the improvement process is the collection of valid data on the actual performance of the practice. The European Society for Quality and Safety in Family Practice, one of the WONCA Europe networks, actually prepares a statement on "Equity, a core dimension of quality of primary care", stressing the importance for all primary care professionals to systematically assess social context, and record basic social information for each patient in the medical record.[169] Not all the problematic points can be addressed at the same time, priority targets should be identified.
- A supportive environment for change is essential: improvement of the organisation of care and the care processes, stimulation of teamwork in multidisciplinary collaboration, provide facilitating measures and infrastructures. Better care is very often associated first of all with more advanced ICT arrangements and presence of interprofessional teams.

When providers of different professions have personal contact, the results are better than when only written interaction is used.

- Quality care is more than linear implementation of guidelines. It is about circular processes where the patient's goals, the context, the scientific professional evidence, the health care system and the team of providers interact, continuously integrating the different dimensions. Finally, it is about the creation of a culture in primary care in which continuous quality improvement at the personal and practice level is a normal component of primary care work. In order to facilitate this cultural change, the traditional Command-and-Control bureaucratic organisational model, should give way for a co-operation, based on "Complex Adaptive System"-models (see Chapter 7).

On 17 August 1585 the Spanish Troops, under the Leadership of Alexander Farnese, Took the City of Antwerp

When looking at quality indicators in Europe, I was amazed by the differences between the Netherlands, the northern Dutch-speaking part of Belgium and the southern French-speaking part of Belgium. I collected data in the nineties that indicated some major differences. Already in 1997 Belgium performed considerably more coronary bypass-surgery interventions than the Netherlands. The number of acute care beds per 1,000 population was 4.6 in Belgium and 3.3. in the Netherlands. In that same year the outpatient antibiotic sales in the Netherlands were 9 defined daily doses per one thousand inhabitants per day, in Belgium it was 27, in France 36. Moreover, the broad-spectrum antibiotics had a much bigger share of the total prescription in Belgium than in the Netherlands, and in France the share was even bigger. When looking at cephalosporins (an antibiotic) Belgium and France used considerably more third and fourth generation cephalosporins than the Netherlands. For different respiratory problems, the prescription rate of antibiotics was systematically higher in Spain than in Denmark.

So, there was a clear European north-south axis in prescription patterns. And also the bacteria knew this: on a north-south axis from Denmark to Spain the "turning point" for antibiotic resistance was in Brussels. The same pattern as for antibiotics was present in consumption of benzodiazepines (tranquillisers). France consumed 3.5 times as many tranquillisers as the Netherlands, but also in Belgium there was a clear difference e.g. between the consumption in people over 45 years in Aalst (Flanders) (20,9% of the population) and Liège (24,9%). The acceptance of a patient list system by family physicians in Flanders was two times the percentage of the French-speaking part of the country. The cost of medical imaging per inhabitant was up to two times as high in the French-speaking part, compared to Flanders. So, there seems to be a kind of north-south axis with Brussels as a "turning point".

In order to better understand the background of this important difference in quality indicators (in antibiotic-prescription, benzodiazepine-prescription, health care organisation,...), I first tried to find a historical explanation. And of course, I came across a historical background of the north-south divide, when discovering that on 17 August 1585 the Spanish troops, under the leadership of Alexander Farnese, took Antwerp and a lot of Flemish intellectuals and higher educated people fled to the Netherlands, leaving the Habsburg empire behind. That event created a clear frontier between the Calvinistic north (the Netherlands) and the Catholic south (the French-speaking part of Belgium, France and Spain). A hypothesis could be that religious differences between Calvinistic and Catholic societies are reflected in health care and health culture. In his book *Die protestantische Ethik und der Geist des Kapitalismus* (1904-05) the German philosopher Max Weber related socio-economic and cultural differences to religious differences.[170] Weber illustrates the differences between Calvinism and Catholicism. Some of those differences may be helpful to understand also the differences in health care and health culture.

In Calvinist societies, according to Weber, the focus is on rationalisation, opposite to the "Catholic superstitions", with magic and ritualism. In Calvinism the focus is on horizontal relationship: as opposed to the medieval Catholic Church, characterised by strict hierarchical distinction between the priest and the layman. In Calvinism the focus is on individual responsibility, whereas in Catholicism the ritual of confession creates the opportunity for rearrangement between God and men. One of the characteristic aspects of popular Catholic devotion was the "pilgrimage". This pilgrimage consisted of visiting one of the numerous sacred places. Most of the time the motivation bears witness to a mentality of instrumental religiosity. The purpose is to touch a sacred image, to turn around a holy object, to bathe in the holy water. And it was crucial to get a devotional picture to take home or sacred water from a local holy source. This was said to have healing effects. With a little bit of imagination, one could make the link with the visit to a tertiary care hospital, looking for healing and bringing a CT scan back home. The instrumental religiosity could be related to the intake of a lot of medication. The focus in this approach was the individual. Mutatis mutandis, in the Calvinist culture the focus is on the collectivity. Transparency and public accountability are central, so you "should" follow the guidelines (EBM). There is no such a thing as "diagnostic and therapeutic freedom", and certainly no possibility for rearrangement by confession. Just as a hypothesis: could it be that in the Netherlands, the fact that less antibiotics are prescribed, is embedded in five centuries of Calvinist culture, focusing on transparency and accountability, whereas in Belgium, and certainly in the French-speaking part, and in France the "colloque singulier" creates the context for prescribing of (broad spectrum) antibiotics (although both physician and patient know that this is not really scientifically sound), but the patient asks for it and the doctor wants to be kind to the patient; and after the consultation the "rearrangement" is possible through the "confession". The Belgian researcher Reginald Deschepper did interviews in a Dutch and a Belgian city on upper respiratory tract diseases and found that the Dutch participants labelled most of these episodes as "common cold" or "flue", whereas the Flemish participants labelled most of their upper respiratory tract episodes as "bronchitis".[171] Moreover, the Flemish participants used more antibiotics. It became clear that participants with a Protestant background were more sceptical about medicines than those with a Catholic background.

Undoubtedly, this kind of research faces difficulties when it comes to conclude about causality. But at least, these hypotheses and small scale findings may stimulate the reflection about the importance of the cultural context when trying to improve quality of care. Of course, the increasing multiculturality in society will reshape the cultural mosaic and its influence on care processes.

Conclusion

Improving quality of health care is a complex challenge. It requires appropriate data, correct analysis of the challenges, exploration of knowledge, skills and attitudes of both providers and patients, and has to integrate medical/ professional evidence with contextual and policy evidence. Moreover, these processes are embedded in cultural contexts reflecting the crossroads of societal change. The approach to care delivery will be based on person-centred interprofessional interactions, creating iterative processes, very often adaptive and versatile, addressing the challenges of societal change.

Reflection by Mieke van Driel

Since the paper on the need for research on quality in primary care was published in *The Lancet* nearly 15 years ago the field of health care and specifically primary health care has evolved. Soaring costs of highly specialised hospital care and increasing complexity of an ageing multi-morbid population are pushing patients out of hospitals into the care of primary care teams, who have become experts in "generalist care".

The quality of care debate is topical, more than ever. The question about best value for money dominates policy agendas all over the world, but how we define best quality of care is shifting. The voice of patients has inspired initiatives such as the Patient-Centred Outcomes Research Institute (PCORI) in the USA, which promotes research measuring outcomes that are relevant to patients. Primary care has welcomed the attention for a more goal-oriented approach to care as it is at the core of general practitioners' clinical practice. Research based on these principles is likely to be more relevant and usable in day-to-day patient care.

However, many challenges remain. Jan De Maeseneer points to the importance of the cultural context and the policy environment as inextricable components of the care process. Lessons from the struggle to curb growing antimicrobial resistance and safeguard antibiotics for the future, show that culture and policy are more powerful drivers than high quality medical evidence. Therefore, understanding and addressing all factors impacting on care and care delivery is vital to achieving better outcomes for patients. The tools required for this more comprehensive view of care with the patient at the centre are increasingly available. The question is how we define and measure success. It is imperative that this debate involves all stakeholders and uses a "co-creation" approach.

Ensuring that best quality care is available to everyone, remains the biggest challenge of all. Even though medical science continues to improve effectiveness of treatments and prevent infectious disease, embarrassing disparities in opportunities for good health still exist worldwide between countries, but also within countries, regions and local areas. In the debate around quality of care, health care equity deserves centre stage. Only then can we genuinely say we are "taking care of quality".

Mieke van Driel, MD, DTM&H, MSc, PhD, FRACGP. Professor of General Practice and Head of the Primary Care Clinical Unit, Faculty of Medicine, University of Queensland, Australia. She also practices as a General Practitioner in an Aboriginal Medical Service. Before moving to Australia in 2008 she completed her PhD studying the gap between evidence and clinical practice, at the Department of Family Medicine and Primary Care, Ghent University, Belgium.

Chapter 7:
Training (Family) Physicians and Health Care Professionals for the 21st Century

Memories of 26 years of professorship...

- Wednesday 18 November 1998: after a long debate a two-third majority of the Faculty Council voted in favour of the new curriculum and approved the reform.
- A Skype interview with a Palestinian young woman with cystic fibrosis, in the first lecture of the first year in medicine. We discussed the difficulties for people living in the Occupied Territories, to access quality health care. Also, medications that this patient needed were not available. Some months later, we were informed that the patient died due to severe complications. The reactions of the students – shock, grieve, anger,... – were remarkable, and the way they communicated their condolences to the Palestinian family was amazing.
- A clinical case discussion with a young woman with multiple sclerosis, exploring the impact the disease had on her life, especially the difficulties she experienced to continue her job and being accepted by the Occupational Medicine physician as a "normal employee".
- The interactive lecture with an undocumented patient from Somalia with a severe chronic illness, who just had received from the Belgian Department of Home Affairs the edict to leave the country within 2 weeks, as he could not be given "refugee status". The only way to overrule this edict was to appeal based on the medical conditions of the person. Three out of four students were in favour of writing an advocacy letter, one out of four was against. The debate that followed touched the essence of what it means to be a doctor.
- The reaction of the students in the debate during the "health economic" course with Professor Lieven Annemans on "Choices in Health Care". The students have to take the role of the Minister of Health, and to select in the framework of a limited additional budget a set of interventions out of a broader menu. Students concluded: "We now understand how difficult the job of our politicians is, and what it means to make choices in health care at national level".
- The supportive interaction in the mentor group when one of the seven students told us that, due to family problems, she had to temporarily interrupt her studies in medicine.
- Wednesday 11 November 2009: Laetitia, Lauren and Emilie, 3 first-year students, were killed in an accident, and students and staff try to cope with this loss in the weeks, months and years after...

The Battle of Crécy (1346)

It is February 1970. As always on Friday morning 8.30 a.m., there is the "history lesson" for the last-year students at secondary school. For the third time in our secondary school trajectory, we are studying the Hundred Years' War and the teacher explains in detail the changing military tactics in medieval warfare. He uses the Battle of Crécy in 1346 between the English and the French to illustrate the dramatic transformation in the character of warfare from antiquity, changing military tactics and the role of cavalry and artillery.

In a meeting with the student council in the week before, we have decided that we would no longer accept to study (for the third time) the medieval problems, but that we wanted to study what actually happened in society, not only in our country, but worldwide. The action strategy was that during the lesson, every minute, one of the students would draw his history book on the ground. After six minutes the teacher understood that something was happening. I was asked by the students to explain, so I took the floor and explained that for us, apart from our knowledge about medieval warfare, it was important to understand what actually happened in our own country, in Vietnam, in the African liberation movements,... From the debate that followed came a proposal by the students: in groups of 5 we would prepare one topic related to the actual situation in the world, the students would give an introduction, and then a debate would follow.

And so it happened, and the teacher afterwards agreed that the class had never learned more on history than during these debates. Later on, in a team under the leadership of my brother Paul, in the framework of "Interschol", a broad movement of secondary school students in Ghent, we developed integrated books that dealt with problems from different angles and could be used in different lessons. One of the books was on the Vietnam War, dealing with the disciplines French, chemistry, biology (on the effects of "Agent Orange"), geography, sociology, anthropology, mathematics,... Other books dealt with Southern Africa, India, Guatemala...

This was my first experience in "curriculum reform", and in those days I was not aware at all, that many other experiences in this field would cross my path in life.

Family Medicine and Primary Care

Involvement in Curriculum Reform as a Student

In March 1974 on the initiative of Professor E. Nihoul, a microbiologist at Ghent University with a lot of interest in curriculum innovation, we had the opportunity to meet with Professor Georges E. Miller, an absolute authority in medical education. He explained us the famous "pyramid", illustrating the difference between "knows" (knowledge), "knows-how" (competence), "shows-how" (performance) and "does" (action).[172] Professor Miller instructed to a group of motivated professors and students how these different components underpin a framework for clinical assessment. During 2 days he evaluated the educational program at the medical faculty and at the end came to the conclusion that there were two major problems: "The first problem was that there were no clear objectives defined for the undergraduate training program, and the second problem was that there was no faculty, i.e. there was no structure where in a systematic way documented decisions about the development of the curriculum could be taken".

In the meantime, I participated in a lot of working parties, revising the curriculum, what mostly was restricted to shifting a discipline from one study year to another, reducing the teaching hours of physics and increasing the teaching hours of histology,...

In the same year we visited the new educational program at Maastricht University in the Netherlands with a group of students, and for the first time in our life, we were confronted with problem-based learning, skills lab training, use of simulated patients,... A completely different world than the one we were trained in.

A Crisis is an Opportunity

In June 1997 I was sitting in the faculty room as head of Department of Family Medicine and Primary Health Care, listening to the conclusions of the "Accreditation Team" of the "Accreditation Organisation of the Netherlands and

Flanders" (NVAO), that for the first time had visited our faculty and assessed the undergraduate medical training program. The conclusions were astonishing: "The program has no clear objectives, there is a lack of integration between basic sciences and clinical sciences, there is almost complete absence of skills training, especially training in doctor-patient communication; the exposure to the patient only starts in the 7th (and last) year of the undergraduate program, there is no appropriate assessment of clinical skills and medical decision making, and absence of any scientific work (no master thesis). There is only one positive point: the contribution that the discipline of family medicine makes to the undergraduate curriculum, providing teaching in patient-centred care, integrated care and exposure to family medicine practices in the community".

The faculty asked me if I wanted to take over the leadership of the Educational Committee from Professor N. Lameire, with the mandate that the next assessment in 2005 should be better. The sense of urgency increased when in October 1998 only 74 students applied for the undergraduate medical training program at Ghent University.

From the very beginning the Educational Committee decided that a "superficial" reform of the curriculum was not the way to go, but that the curriculum should be reconstructed from scratch. Moreover, it was important that all stakeholders would be involved in the reform process, and especially the need for participation by the students was emphasised. In order not to reinvent the wheel, the faculty decided to visit curricula abroad that already had demonstrated their innovative strengths: Maastricht, Nijmegen (both in the Netherlands), Toronto, McMaster University, University of Sherbrooke, McGill University (Canada) enabled the Committee to understand what could be the innovations appropriate for Ghent University. A vision document on "The physician for the 21st century" indicated clearly that a new type of providers was needed, who were able to interact appropriately with the patient, who had the knowledge, skills and attitude, enabling them to provide high quality care, who were able to function as "reflective practitioners", as scientific scholars, and who could provide the leadership and advocacy to function in a changing health care environment. In 1992 Charles Boelen, Chief Medical Officer for the World Health Organisation's Program on Educational Development for Human Resources, defined the ideal profile of a doctor for the society. The doctor should possess "a mix of aptitudes needed to carry out the range of services that health settings must deliver to meet the requirements of relevance, quality, cost-effectiveness and equity in health".[173] Awareness of important public health issues, ability to use an interdisciplinary approach to solve problems, and adequate communication skills all contribute to becoming a "Five-Star Doctor".[174] Moreover, factors such as living conditions, income, family status, occupation and social environment have serious impact on health, and doctors must take them into account when interacting with a patient.

The vision was translated in a set of learning outcomes, that exactly defined the level that should be reached during the undergraduate training, describing the "product" of this training as a doctor who is able to start a postgraduate training program, either in family medicine, or in one of the specialty disciplines or in preventive or social medicine or in research. In a set of interdisciplinary meetings, a debate about the level of knowledge and skills that should be acquired in relation to different topics, was defined. The Committee decided to make a fundamental switch from a discipline based curriculum with disciplines like chemistry, biology, physics, anatomy, pathology, diagnosis and treatment,... as building blocks towards an integrated contextual medical curriculum, composed of "units", "lines" and with an open mind towards societal developments and social accountability. The "units" were interdisciplinary modules from 4 to 6 weeks, dealing with a topic in an integrated way. The first units dealt with the "Cell" and "Health & Society", then followed by units looking at "Tissue" and "Systems".

The four "lines" create a continuum of learning throughout the whole curriculum. The first line is the **P-line** "problem solving". In this line students learn to search for information, they learn scientific critical appraisal of literature, acquire the basics of statistical analysis in a medical context, are introduced to scientific work, learn medical decision-making and problem-solving (in "tutorials"), and from the third year onwards they learn to deal with clinical problems, first through vignettes, then in case discussions with real patients. In this line, they also learn to deal with uncertainty and to reflect on the limits of medical diagnosis (see Chapter 4) and therapy (see Chapter 5). In the **E-line** "Exploration and Ethics" students explore the organisation of the Belgian health system, they learn about health care in the community (primary health care, nursing homes, other community based services), in a group they produce a policy paper that translates a scientific report into a concrete policy proposal, and in the field of ethics they progressively learn the principles and practice of ethical reasoning. The curriculum also increasingly emphasises interprofessional training. In the master years, students from different training programs (medicine, health promotion, nursing, pharmacy, management,...) develop an interprofessional strategic care plan focusing on a chronic condition with special attention for the multi-morbidity context. Finally, the "studium generale" invites students during the first 4 years of the training to participate actively in at least 3 debates on actual societal and cultural topics like the situation of refugees, choices in health care, global health,... In the 5th year, there is an exercise on "Medical Humanities", where students approach a topic e.g. access to health care, the position of mentally ill in society,... not starting from medical scientific literature, but starting from an exposition, a book, a movie, a play,... In the **V-line** "Communication, Clinical Diagnostic and Therapeutic Skills", the students progressively acquire communication skills, beginning with the exploration of the need of the patient, and ending with complex communicative situations, like breaking bad news, intercultural communication,...[175] The total communication training takes more than 50 hours and is mainly built on small group training, using simulated patients. The clinical skills training starts from the examination of the "normal" and progressively integrates elements of pathology. Finally, students perform integrated consultations with simulated patients. By doing so, they are prepared to take maximal advantage of their clerkships from the fifth year onwards. The **Z-line** "Scientific Work" starts in the first year with writing a scientific paper on a topic in relation to "Health and Society" (psychology, sociology, anthropology, health promotion, social determinants,...), based on 5 articles. In the second year they take a biomedical topic and write another 5-pages paper, and from the third year onwards they prepare for the master thesis, with an exercise in data analysis and producing a statistical report.

The learning is problem-oriented, with in the first years an emphasis on the "normal" functioning, and in the following years the focus switches to the study of health problems, symptoms and complaints, diseases. For the didactic implementation the option is to go for a "mixed method didactic approach", blending traditional lectures (no more than 8 a week), self-directed learning, interactive sessions, clinical case presentations, multi-disciplinary panels, problem-oriented teaching and exposure to clinical reality (observational clerkships). The new curriculum could take advantage of the fact that since 1998 an "entrance examination" at the level of the region of Flanders made sure that the students had acquired a critical level in mathematics, physics, chemistry, and biology. Moreover, the examination also assessed the understanding of communicative interaction and the skills in critical reading.

The Ghent-curriculum devotes special attention to "Community Orientation". In the second and the third year students have to regularly follow and visit a family where a baby was born, observing the development of the baby (physical, psychomotor and psychological) and exploring the context of the family where the child is living in. In the second year, students participate in an interprofessional Community Oriented Primary Care experience (see Chapter 2), where during one week they work in a deprived neighbourhood in the city of Ghent or in other cities and villages. On Monday morning, after having been introduced to the history of the neighbourhood, they visit a socially vulnerable family, and then explore the living context and living conditions in the community. They perform interviews with three primary care providers (family doctors, nurses, social workers, dieticians, pharmacists, informal care givers,...) who are involved in the care of that family. The interviews open their eyes for the importance of social determinants of health, and start the reflection on the context of health and disease. On Tuesday afternoon they bring all the information from their visits together and try to make a "Community Diagnosis". At that moment the confrontation of different perspectives (medical students, nursing students, sociology students, health promotion students,...) sometimes leads to a "clash of cultures", and enables students to frame their own ideas in a broader perspective. Starting from the Community Diagnosis, that is no longer formulated in terms of diseases, but as societal problems (dealing with multiculturality, unemployment, unsafe environments, unhealthy housing conditions, insufficient opportunities for leisure in the community,...) the students formulate possible actions that could address the problems they discovered. At this moment, they confront their ideas with experienced community workers, who help them to make a "reality check". The week ends with fundamental reflections on their role as future health care providers, and with the writing of an advocacy letter to an agency that may improve the living conditions of the family they visited.

From the assessment of this experience we learned that this Community-Oriented Primary Care exercise helps to understand the broader context of health and illness in society, learns the students to appreciate co-operation with other disciplines and motivates them to address upstream causes (social determinants) of ill health[176] (see Chapter 2). Some students report: "It was after that experience that I decided to become a family physician".

The first years of the undergraduate training put special emphasis on exposure to family medicine and primary care: an interview of a family physician with a young patient with cystic fibrosis is used as an introduction to the study of the "Cell". So, whilst students are studying regulatory mechanisms in the cell, illustrated with the condition of cystic fibrosis, they can link it with a real patient that they have seen and listened to. A clerkship in a "nursing home" (year 1) and with a family physician (year 2) further contribute to exposure to primary care.

The curriculum also puts special attention on scientific work. Motivated students, from the second year onwards, can engage in scientific work in research groups or laboratories and acquire 15 ECTS-study points (European Credit Transfer System) extra in the framework of the "Honours Program in the Life Sciences". By doing so, the students are stimulated for research careers. Another Honours Program invites students to participate in innovation of education, creating opportunities to contribute to education improvement. From the third year onwards all students engage in a master thesis, which they defend publically at the end of the first semester of the 5th year.

During their undergraduate curriculum two thirds of the students have an international experience in a European country or overseas in countries like Bolivia, Ecuador, Nicaragua, Uganda, Mozambique, Kenya, Rwanda, Iran, India, Cambodia, Cuba, South-Africa,...

In 2012 the Federal Government decided that the undergraduate training should be shortened from 7 years to 6 years, which required a second fundamental curriculum reform. The Educational Committee took advantage of this reform, to optimise the integration (both horizontal and vertical) in the curriculum, and to introduce the "mentor groups" in the framework of the E-line: groups of 7 students who are during the 6 years under the guidance of an experienced medical staff member and reflect 4 times a year about their evolution to become medical professionals.[177] The first cohort of this new program will graduate in 2018, but there is actually already so much evidence that this has contributed a lot to personal professional development of our students. Moreover, the system functions very well in early detection of students who have problems during

Family Medicine and Primary Care

their training program, and this approach allows early intervention, illustrating that the academic staff "takes care" of the students.

From the first day, a group of motivated professors and many students contributed actively to the development of the new curriculum, and the students' ownership was clear: "It is OUR curriculum". The ownership by the teaching staff took more time, but gradually increased, especially because more than 100 academic staff members contributed in "working groups" and "committees" to the new project. A convincing factor was that a lot of professors saw their children study medicine in the "new curriculum" and observed the difference and improvement.

2005: a First Assessment of the New Undergraduate Curriculum

An international "Accreditation Commission" visited the new training program at Ghent University during 3 days in 2005. The report of the Commission was extremely positive[178] and recognised that there were clear objectives in relation to the required competencies. There was a systematic development of the new curriculum, and the system of working with "units" and "lines" was highly appreciated. The role of the central steering by the Educational Committee was appreciated. The Commission recognised that there was special emphasis on scientific orientation, clinical competence and societal relevance. Moreover, the undergraduate medical training program at Ghent University was the first program at the University to receive a "Special Quality Award" for its "Community Orientation and Social Accountability", and the Commission concluded that the program gives "a very relevant focus to the social accountability in an excellent way". According to the "Accreditation Commission", the project "Community-Oriented Primary Care" emphasises the need to understand social functioning and "this project is, from an international perspective, a unique way of dealing with social context in the training of future physicians".

This positive evaluation, together with a continuously increasing number of students applying for the undergraduate training program at Ghent University

(361 in 2016), contributed to the fact that the Faculty of Medicine and Health Sciences decided to continue the process of innovation and improvement of the curriculum.

Apart from the external accreditation procedure, it was important to assess the impact of the new curriculum on learning styles and knowledge acquisition. The students of the newly integrated contextual curriculum showed more structuring of subject matter by integrating different aspects into a whole.[179] Moreover, the new medical curriculum had a significant impact on acquiring processing strategies, regulation strategies, and on learning orientations. The clear built-up of the curriculum and vertical and horizontal integration of subject knowledge seemed to have significantly reduced the lack of integration and promoted at an earlier stage structuring, relating critical processing and vocational orientation.[180] For many professors in the faculty, however, the most important concern was the impact of the transition from the conventional to the integrated contextual medical curriculum on knowledge acquisition. It became clear that a stronger integration of biomedical and clinical sciences in the curriculum leads to a more gradual and steady mastery of clinical knowledge. Consistently, the students in the new curriculum reflect a significantly larger mastery. At the same time, a stronger emphasis on clinical relevant biomedical sciences in the early years of the new curriculum was related with a steeper learning curve of basic biomedical knowledge. This type of knowledge continues to increase in the later years of the curriculum.[181] So, in summary, both in learning styles and in outcomes, as far as knowledge is concerned, the aims of the curriculum reform were achieved. Moreover, a lot of qualitative information, from the preceptors that compared the performance during the clerkships in the hospitals of the "conventional" and the "new" curriculum students, documented that the training program at Ghent University manages to train "a new type of physician".

The students played an essential role in the whole process of curriculum change. They were active from the first day, contributed to the concept papers, participated in the Educational Committee meetings and in the Commissions that prepared the different "units and lines". During the whole process they acted as "information hubs" and critical reflectors and made a lot of very positive proposals in the different phases, especially in the implementation phase. Since 2005 they have been investing a complete week of their holidays to reflect with representatives of all study years on the strong and weak points of the curriculum, and have been formulating proposals for improvement. Each year this has led to a report (often 30 to 40 pages) that details their proposals and is presented annually in the meeting of the Educational Committee of October. The topics of the report fill in the "Quality monitoring agenda" of the Educational Committee. To have a well-structured and strong student participation, as realised in Ghent by the Student Workgroup In Medical Education, is an asset for a Faculty of Medicine and Health Sciences.[182]

Finally, curriculum management is of utmost importance and the success of the new curriculum was the consequence of a group of very committed "curriculum managers". When I ended my career as chair of the Educational Committee on the 1st of October 2016, a new leadership took over: a basic scientist, an ENT-surgeon and a family physician. Integrating theory and clinical experience from the first year of the Master-program and strengthening the ICT-component of the learning process are their next challenges.

The Master-after-Master Interuniversity Training Program in Family Medicine

As indicated earlier, already in 1997, at the first assessment, the important contribution of the Department of Family Medicine and Primary Health Care in the undergraduate curriculum was recognised. This contribution originated from the experience that started in 1984 when the 4 Flemish universities decided to create one common postgraduate training program in family medicine (see Chapter 1 and 10). That program was built on innovative educational principles, starting from a list of competencies and translating them into appropriate didactic approaches. The strength of the Interuniversity Centre for Family Medicine Training was that the 4 heads of department of family medicine were really willing to co-create and made an effort to make the training program in concordance with the European Directives that from 1986 onwards orientated family medicine training in Europe. After a complex transition period, where the 7th year of the undergraduate training also was "integrated" in the family medicine training program, finally the decree of 5 April 1995 established a 2-years interuniversity postgraduate training after the 7 years' undergraduate program. In 2018 the family medicine master-after-master program will be extended from 2 to 3 years: 2 and a half years in two training practices in family medicine, 6 months in a hospital, according to the European Directive. The co-operation between the four departments in Flanders remains the cornerstone of successful developments, especially through the sharing of "training practices". These developments contributed to the academic profiling of the discipline of family medicine, but to a large extent also influenced the political debate about the role and function of primary health care in Flanders. The fact that more than 1,000 practices will be, from 2020 onwards, involved in the training of future family physicians, illustrates the impact academic departments can have. Moreover, the heads of department regularly participated in the societal and political debate on the future of family medicine and primary health care, e.g. when they published the report "Together We Change" in December 2014 (see Chapter 8), that set the foundation for the primary health care policy as defined at the Flemish primary care conference in 2017.

The most important contribution family medicine made to the improvement of the training of future health professionals, was the development of innovative educational approaches for "Workplace Learning". Giving feedback, critical reflective practice, implementation of Evidence-Based Medicine, focusing on the goals of the patient,... were underpinned with appropriate didactic tools. These insights were later translated towards training of health professionals in hospitals and in other settings. In 2005 an "Accreditation Committee" assessed the training program in family medicine in Flanders.[183] The assessment was very positive about the way the training program was organised but emphasised the need for more orientation towards scientific work. The implementation of Evidence-Based Medicine was appropriate and the didactics innovative, with special emphasis on E-learning. Moreover, the participation of all stakeholders (staff, preceptors, students,...) was highly appreciated. Besides this global positive assessment, this training program was awarded with a Special Quality Award for the "Impact of the network organisation and the societal impact of the co-operation between the 4 departments of family medicine". The report commented that this interuniversity network organisation could be a model for other training programs in different disciplines in medicine. The training in the family medicine program illustrates how, despite too limited resources, an academic training program of high quality can be put into practice. The challenge today is to scale up this program in order to train sufficient numbers to address increasing needs, due to the demographical and epidemiological transition.

In order to scale up the training capacity in Flanders, there was a need to reconstruct the actual payment-relationship between preceptors and trainees in family medicine. Since 2009 all the trainees have been employed by a not-for-profit organisation, and the preceptor has been able to focus on the pedagogical role.

The search for a New Professionalism

In order to be "socially accountable", training programs for health professionals' education should be informed by a broad group of stakeholders who are able to contribute to the formulation of new "professional profiles" that will be needed in health care and welfare in the future to respond to societal change. In Flanders (Belgium), the Strategic Advisory Board for Welfare,[184] Health and Family, composed of 28 stakeholders from the large civil society: representatives of the supply – and the demand-side, representatives of the labour forces in the sector of wellbeing, health and family; professionals; socio-economic organisations (trade unions, employers,...); representatives of specific societal groups (e.g. people living in poverty,...) and independent experts formulated a vision statement on "new professionalism". The Board started from an analysis of the changing society, characterised by more complexity with an increasing ethnic and cultural diversity, an economic trend toward more competition, an aging society, a change in family structures, increasing chronic conditions and scientific and technological developments.

Traditionally, the answers to these challenges have been sought in more specialisation (in a strategy to "reduce complexity"), instrumentalisation of professional work and "medicalisation and therapeutisation".

The Board formulated the vision that new answers are needed: a more generalist approach is required and emphasis should be on connecting people: "Connectedness as a pre-condition for autonomy". In order to achieve these goals professionals require more generalist competencies: enabling a professional to provide care and support based on a generalist strategy or approach, with the aim to address a broad range of unspecified health and/or well-being (related) problems. The care should focus on quality of life, on supporting self-care and care of informal care-givers, strengthen social cohesion, embracing diversity and appropriate use of technology and ICT.

The "new professionals" should pay attention to functional status, pay attention to what really matters for people, support autonomy through information and strengthen participation and inclusion. Moreover, the Board did not see the solution to the challenges in the creation of a "super-professional", but in stimulating interprofessional co-operation.

This vision statement was unanimously approved by all the stakeholders and is translated to change processes, both in training and in organisation of care at the workplace.

Broadening the Scope: Health Professional Education in an International Perspective

Professor Anselme Derese, colleague at the department, explored in the late nineties the possibility for international co-operation on innovation of health professional education. He came across an organisation named: "The Network: Towards Unity for Health" (http://thenetworktufh.org/). This organisation was founded in 1979 at a meeting in Kingstone, Jamaica, where a group of academics from all over the world started a network focusing on innovative approaches to health professional education in the framework of "Community-Oriented Educational Institutions". Thanks to the co-operation with the World Health Organisation the membership increased with a lot of universities and organisations from developing countries and non-governmental organisations from all continents. One of the founding institutions was Maastricht University (the Netherlands), that took responsibility for the secretariat. A peer-reviewed journal "*Education for Health*" (www.educationforhealth.net) created a platform for publication of innovative approaches like problem-based learning, patient-oriented medical education, community-based education,... The annual conferences were an opportunity that was picked up at Ghent University, and the Faculty of Medicine became a member in 1995. In 2002, The Network: TUFH became a NGO "in official relationship with WHO". The contributions by the staff from Ghent University at conferences in the period 2001-2003 resulted in an invitation to organise the annual world conference at Ghent University in 2006 on the topic "Increasing social accountability of health professional education". Thanks to a grant by the university, Sara Willems, who just finished a PhD on "The socio-economic gradient in health: a never-ending story"[45] (see Chapter 2), was able to take the co-ordination of this conference. Over 300 people from more than 40 countries attended the meetings.

In 2007 I was elected Secretary General of "The Network: Towards Unity for Health", and the Department of Family Medicine and Primary Health Care took over the secretariat from Maastricht University. What made The Network an inspiring organisation was the fact that at the meetings all the participants had "a story to tell" on how they made their training programs more relevant to the needs of their populations, how they engaged with local communities, not only for teaching purposes, but to work together to improve local health conditions. The important participation of staff and students from low- and middle-income countries contributed to the "global" dimension of the organisation. In the period 2007-2015 The Network: Towards Unity for Health evolved more and more towards a "Network of networks", co-operating with organisations like Global Health through Education Training and Service (www.ghets.org), the Consortium of Longitudinal Integrated Clerkships (CLIC http://www.clicmeded.com), the "Training for Health Equity Network" (THEnet: http://thenetcommunity.org),... The "Training for Health Equity Network" especially emphasised the need for recruitment of students, coming from minority groups, socially deprived areas,... in order to address the needs of those communities. In 2011 Ghent University became one of the 11 schools of the Training for Health Equity Network.

THEnet produced a monograph, "THEnet's Evaluation Framework for Socially Accountable Health Professional Educations", that can be used to assess the following questions: how does a school work? What do we do? What difference do we make in our efforts to make the health professionals we train more fit to respond to the needs of the community?[185] The topic of "social accountability" was also at the centre of the World Summit On Social Accountability: Improving the Impact of Education Institutions on People's Health and of the "Tunis

Declaration" launched on 12 April 2017 in a meeting chaired by the Minister of Health of Tunisia and attended by representatives of Institutions for Health Professional Education from 45 countries. The Tunis Declaration clearly states its belief that the commitments of its participants and partners will result in measurable improvement in societies' priority health needs, sustainable environmental health and the well-being of all people, through the action plan centred on four strategic axes:

- expanding information, communication and advocacy to promote social accountability in partnerships embracing academic and educational institutions, governments, professional associations, managers, and communities;
- ensuring the development of the knowledge, skills and attitudes required for social accountable practice in the education of future health workers;
- accreditation founded on the principles of social responsibility is an obligation for all faculties of medicine and schools of health to enhance their impact on the health of society;
- using a systematic approach involving the political and the socio-economic worlds to develop ethical and equitable intercultural partnerships and health alliances.

The Need for Interprofessional Education

In 2012 the "Global Forum on Innovation in Health Professional Education" started in the framework of the National Academies of Sciences, Engineering and Medicine (Washington, USA). The Forum brings together stakeholders from multiple nations and professions to network and discuss on issues within health professional education. Actually, there are 56 members appointed representing 19 different disciplines from 9 countries. Since 2012 I am a member of the Global Forum.

The Forum has dealt with a lot of important issues, like "assessing health professional education", "building health workforce capacity through community-based health professional education", "exploring the role of accreditation in enhancing quality and innovation in health professionals education",... The Forum has a strong emphasis on interprofessional education for collaboration.[183]

In order to prepare health care students in a practice-ready way, the education they receive should mirror the reality of the health care context they will enter after graduation. The actual context of older patients with chronic diseases and multi-morbidity requires interprofessional collaboration in order to provide high quality patient care. The growing complexity of the health care delivery context, through the introduction of new health care disciplines and services, requires a curriculum where students from different professional backgrounds learn with, from and about each other. As such, and in line with the report of the 2010 Lancet Commission, interprofessional education (IPE) can be seen as a tool to create linkages between the educational system and the health care delivery system.[97] IPE as an operationalisation of the interdependency of both worlds provides opportunities to achieve the quadruple aim: better patient care, better population health, more efficient and affordable educational and health care systems and finally improving the work life of health care providers[58] (see Chapter 8). To achieve these outcomes an IPE curriculum should be soundly based in an interprofessional competency framework, and thoroughly evaluated, both at student level and at curriculum level.[186]

IPE also has a transformative component leading to the acquisition of leadership skills needed by providers when entering the complex health care system. The learning continuum stretches from the undergraduate level, through the graduate level, into the lifelong learning continuum. Fundamental in health care education are patient contacts, equally so in IPE. As Osler said: "He who studies medicine without books sails an uncharted sea, but he who studies medicine without patients does not go to sea at all".[187] Here is where workplace learning comes in. Traineeships are a fortiori important in IPE where health care providers (students or practitioners) care for the same patient. Family physicians for instance co-operating with expert palliative care nurses in palliative care at home learn a lot about physical and psychosocial symptom management both from the nurses and from the patients through listening, observing, discussion and joint reflection.[188] At the same time the expert nurses report equal learning during collaboration with family physicians, indicating the reciprocity of workplace learning. Introducing IPE during undergraduate education can prepare health care providers to share their competences and to acknowledge each other's expertise. This leads to better collaboration in practice, and in turn, leads to a lifelong interprofessional workplace learning curriculum.

To inform us on the educational formats and didactical techniques during undergraduate education and to gain full insight into the mechanisms of the lifelong interprofessional learning curriculum we can draw on complexity science.[189] Looking at learning communities and health care teams as Complex Adaptive Systems (CAS) allows us to apply the complexity science principles into the educational context. Some examples:

- Individuals within a system are independent and can act autonomously: self-directed experiential learning is an efficient learning process;
- The behaviour of an individual in a system evolves according to feedback upon its actions: immediate observed feedback informs the learning which is social and relational in nature;
- Interactions between individuals can produce non-linear and unpredictable results: the learning curve of students during traineeship can evolve fast or slow, more or less steep in an unpredictable way;
- A system is co-evolving with its environment: transformative learning goes beyond the competence level and reaches the capability level, where individuals are able to adapt to change, generate new knowledge, and continue to improve their performance.

That is what is needed in order to deliver health care providers able to function in VUCA-times (Volatile, Uncertain, Complex, Ambiguous) both as clinicians and as clinical leaders.[190] Next to the applicability of complexity science insights for the understanding of learning, the same principles can also be used to inform the management of organisations, be it educational institutions in designing curricula or health care teams and organisations in delivering health care.[191] In a bureaucratic management structure roles are being strictly defined, while in a CAS-environment much more attention is being paid to the relationship building between individuals. In a management structure focus is more on knowledge, while in a CAS learning as tool for evolution is more on the foreground. In a bureaucratic management structure Command-and-Control is rather strict, while in a CAS accepting uncertainty and paradox leads to stimulation of improvisation and input from individuals. Managing an organisation according to the CAS-principles allows for more self-organisation and adaptiveness to rapidly changing environments, fundamental aspects when it comes to learning in this era.

Reinventing the University in the 21st Century

The switch towards more interdisciplinary work and interprofessional education requires a fundamental rethinking of the way universities are organised.

One can wonder whether "faculties" are still an appropriate way to organise a university? Indeed, most of the universities worldwide are structured in faculties, some of which originated in medieval times. Today, it is obvious that progress in science and education transgresses the borders of a discipline and of a faculty. The example of neurosciences illustrates that spear point research requires the co-operation of at least three "faculties": medicine, psychology, engineering...

There is no doubt that modern universities actually try to stimulate interdisciplinary research and education, but frequently the spirit of "medieval guilds" dominates the need for open co-operation. Moreover, although most of the financial sponsors preach the newspeak of interdisciplinarity, the reality of financial regulations may be a bottleneck.

Why should we not think about a fundamentally other type of organisation? Could a university not be based on groups that develop a set of overarching "competencies, capacities and capabilities"? E.g. a "capacity group" on "brain-behaviour-movement-imaging" that on the one hand stimulates the shared use of technology (e.g. functional MRI) and on the other hand guarantees interdisciplinary thinking and formulating research questions, from the very beginning. This approach prevents researchers from over-focusing ("to know almost everything about almost nothing"). Another "capacity group" could work on "communication-learning-transfer". Another group could deal with "structure, process and outcome of human interventions" (involving history, economy, anthropology, sociology, ethics, philology, geography,...). These capacity groups could engage their staff in flexible project groups that work on research projects (both within and between capacity groups) and other project groups that engage in teaching (teaching being a dynamic project and not a predefined "task").

Research domains like environmental sciences make clear that a continuous interaction between basic sciences and so-called "applied sciences" is needed. Moreover, contextualisation of research will prevent universities from overlooking important dimensions of research results like affordability, accessibility, acceptability, sustainability,... Would it not be a good idea to end every PhD thesis with a final chapter on "societal relevance/impact"?

The actual assessment of research output with the system of "impact-factors" is highly inappropriate.[192] There are important biases: discipline bias, regional bias,... Moreover, one could question the link between the impact factor of a journal and the quality of published research, as only a limited amount of published articles contributes to the "impact-factor" of a certain journal. Perhaps the idea of exploring also the "societal" impact of research could be worthwhile.[193] It could prevent us from too reductionist approaches, bearing in mind that "not everything that is countable, counts and not everything that counts, is countable" (Isaac Newton).

This chapter described the need for rethinking the education, and how this worked in the fundamental reform of the undergraduate medical curriculum at Ghent University. However, there are important threats to university education. The first one has to do with the increasing "flexibilisation" of the educational process. On the one hand, this may have advantages for specific groups of students (e.g. students that combine work with studies), on the other hand it creates a mentality of "a master degree is the end of a process where the student, as in the supermarket, just adds the different credits to his/her basket", overlooking the fact that learning is fundamentally a "social process and needs interaction with peers". Moreover, the increasing "juridification" of the professor-student relationship may hinder the realisation of creative forms of teaching and assessment, because it becomes impossible to integrate them in "juridically safe" procedures, so that reductionist (quantitative) approaches replace qualitative processes of development, encouragement and trust-building.

Finally, also the organisational model of universities, reflects too much the "Command-and-Control" bureaucratic model. These approaches don't work in an academic environment and the risk of ending up in a "meritocratic reductionist system" is obvious. A functional approach towards career development, with clear goals, formulated at the level of groups and inviting all the group members to contribute seems to be an option for innovative human resources management. However, it remains difficult to reconcile the managerial need for "figures and data" with the typical requirements of an academic environment. So, also our universities could be inspired by the "Complex Adaptive System" approach that could open new perspectives: replacing strict "role defining" by "building relationships", "tight structuring" by "loose coupling", "simplifying" by "complicating", "socialising" by "diversifying", "decision-making" by "sense-making", "knowing" by "learning", "controlling" by "improvising" and "planning based on forecasting" by "thinking about the future".

The fundamental question is: will universities be able to adopt the required transformative power to contribute to a better future for the people and the planet?

Reflection by Charles Boelen

In our world of globalisation and hyperspecialisation we run a risk of rewarding pieces of a mosaic more than the entire mosaic and what it represents. Similarly, in the health sector, an organ and disease oriented offer of service may prevail on a whole person oriented one. Also, immediate expectations of individuals may conflict with long-term expectations of the entire society. In contrast, the implementation of the concept of social accountability should prevent from these counterproductive divides and be the catalyst of a reconciliation. Indeed, social accountability entails a triple obligation: the identification of our current and future health challenges; the mobilisation of creative minds in education, research and service provision to address these challenges; and the commitment that operated changes will produce the highest possible impact on people's well-being. If demonstrated by the University, such coherence and unity of purpose may facilitate the emergence of an equitable, efficient and sustainable health system.

Among key health stakeholders, the University has the potential to lead a fundamental transformational process in the health sector. For this, its credibility must rely on a vision inspired by society's needs, on the capacity to consult and interact with other stakeholders, on the courage to experiment and disseminate alternative models of health service. With this prerequisite, it should be able to prepare a health workforce of a different kind, it should foster alliances with other constituencies for a system approach on health determinants, it should have the ear of policy-makers to build a happier society.

Dr Charles Boelen
International consultant in health system and personnel
Former co-ordinator of the World Health Organisation (Headquarters in Geneva) program of human resources for health

Chapter 8:

Policy Change: from Care for Individuals and Families towards Accountability for a Population

1 September 1983. Hundreds of enthusiastic pupils leaving the school and crossing the street in front of the Community Health Centre Botermarkt. All of a sudden a car hits one of the pupils walking on the pedestrian crosswalk. The boy is heavily wounded and one of the teachers who observed the accident runs into the CHC to ask for our assistance. The nurse and myself are examining the victim, laying down at the street but fortunately the "vital signs" are okay. An ambulance is called and we provide the first aid. The boy is transferred to the hospital.

This was the second severe accident with a pedestrian in one month at the same location.

The community was shocked by this incident and asked for action. With the Community Health Centre we brought together all the stakeholders involved in a Community-Oriented Primary Care approach (see Chapter 2): schools, youth organisations, organisations for the elderly (for whom the crossing also turned out to be very dangerous), local police, the city's Department on Traffic and Infrastructure,... In the first meeting, attended by 40 people, it became obvious that cars were driving too fast and the pedestrian crossing was unsafe, as the road had 2 tracks in each direction. Inhabitants of the neighbourhood were involved in the design of a new project for the road infrastructure and over 500 people participated in a survey proposing different solutions. Finally, a proposal was formulated to the city council and approved. It took 3 years before implementation was finalised, but ever since there have been no major accidents involving pedestrians at this place...

March 2013. I'm sitting near the window on the train on my way to a meeting in Brussels, and I see a lady with a newspaper at the opposite side of the train compartment. She is observing me and asks: "Are you Dr De Maeseneer?" "Yes, I am, how come you know me?" She breaks out in tears and says: "30 years ago, you saved my brother's life." She was the sister of the schoolboy that was severely injured and transferred to the hospital in 1983. She told me that her brother was doing well after a long period of recovery and survived without disabilities. He is a teacher and has a family with 2 children now.

As primary care providers at the crossroads of society and health care, we have the privilege to make a difference both for individuals and communities.

Physicians May Not Go on Strike...

After the Alma-Ata Declaration (see Chapter 1) many countries tried to put the principles of primary care into practice. In Belgium, however, on 21 December 1979 doctors went on strike against the government because they did not agree with the proposed measures to cut some expenses in health care and to limit the "diagnostic and therapeutic freedom" that was in those days very important, in the absence of Evidence Based Medicine with almost no accountability from the side of the providers. With a group of young and progressive doctors, we decided that although a debate about change in the health care system was needed, a strike, where the patient is always the victim, was ethically not acceptable. So we organised a "Committee for Continuity of Care" that could count on an important group of family physicians and specialist doctors who did not participate in this strike movement. The conservative trade unions of doctors ended the strike on 18 January 1980, without obtaining "any results". In the aftermath of this conflict I took the lead of an "Organisation for a Progressive Health Policy" that formulated the platform for the development of primary health care. On 14 December 1980 the following action points were agreed upon:

- the need to start up gatekeeping by the family physicians, with no direct access to specialist care (referral system);
- the need for the creation of global payment systems like capitation for primary care providers;
- establishment of multidisciplinary co-operatives with family physicians, nurses, social workers, co-operating in teams;
- participation of the population in the development of primary care;
- increase of resources for primary care and optimisation of the use of technical resources in secondary care.

Unfortunately, these ideas did not reach the political debate, as the government continued to negotiate with the traditional conservative trade unions of doctors. In the absence of a clear primary care oriented policy, a lot of bottom-up initiatives were taken by groups of providers, together with patient groups, movements from the socio-cultural sector,... In 1982 a first achievement led to the instauration of the possibility for a capitation system (see Chapter 9). In the same year the (regional) Flemish Minister for Health Policy installed

Family Medicine and Primary Care

a "Working Group on Primary Health Care" in order to formulate a plan for "horizontal co-operation of the core disciplines in primary health care". On 23 June 1983 the Working Group published its report, advocating the stimulation of interprofessional co-operation at the primary care level involving family physicians, nurses, home carers, social workers,... in order to provide patient-oriented care.[194] The working party described the bottlenecks that could hinder this development: organisational bottlenecks at the macro, meso and micro level, the need for "models" and the lack of appropriate methodologies; juridical problems (e.g. information-sharing and the privacy of the patient); financial bottlenecks in the framework of the fee-for-service payment system; bottlenecks due to the inappropriate training programs for providers and the need for a change of culture both at the population's and provider's side. Finally, the working group formulated the advice to the Minister to create a "Flemish Institute for Primary Health Care", that should coordinate the activities of the different stakeholders in order to develop a primary care system. Nothing happened with these recommendations and the working group was disbanded. At the regional level some rather isolated initiatives were taken, e.g. supporting multidisciplinary discussions about complex patients in the home care, initiatives for health promotion in the community.

In the meantime at the federal level the "Global Medical Record" was established (see Chapter 1), linking patients to family practices (1990-2002), and a law on "Patient Rights" was voted by the Parliament in 2002, strengthening the position of patients in the care process. In 2006, the Flemish Health Council repeated that strengthening primary care would be necessary to address the challenges of the changing demographical and epidemiological field, especially the increase of chronic conditions and multi-morbidity. These viewpoints were echoed at a big Flemish conference on primary care in 2010, and a symposium in 2013. However, the insights were at that moment not translated in structural changes in the health care system.

Academics Take the Initiative to Change Health Policy

In December 2014, for the first time the four heads of Department of Family Medicine and Primary Health Care at the four Flemish universities presented a report "Together We Change: Primary Health Care Now More Than Ever!".[195] With 3 other Flemish professors: Professor Bert Aertgeerts (KU Leuven), Professor Roy Remmen (University of Antwerp), Professor Dirk Devroey (Free University of Brussels), we described the challenges for the health care system in the 21st century, and formulated proposals for a fundamental change of the primary health care system. This approach was in line with the report "Health 2020: European Policy Framework and Strategy for the 21st Century".[196] This report concluded: "Health 2020 remains committed to a primary health care approach as a corner stone of health systems in the 21st century. Primary Health Care can respond to today's needs by fostering and enabling an environment for partnerships to thrive and encouraging people to participate in new ways in their treatment and take better care of their own health. Making full use of 21st century tools and innovations, such as communication technology – digital records, telemedicine and e-Health – and social media, can contribute to better and more cost-effective care. Recognising patients as a resource and as partners, and being accountable for patient outcomes are important principles". Nowadays, strong primary care should contribute to the realisation of the "Quadruple Aim", i.e. the following 4 goals of the health care system:[61]

- improving the health of the population
- improving patient experience
- reducing cost (in the European approach: "Increasing the 'values' with the resources available")
- improving the work life of health care providers, including clinicians and staff

Challenges for Health Care in the 21st Century

The actual challenges for health care systems worldwide can be summarised as follows:

- **Demographical and epidemiological** developments: we live longer (in 2016 the average life expectancy in the European Union was 84.6 years for men and 89.1 for women). Older age is related to an increase in the prevalence of cancer. Thanks to the improved therapy cancer becomes a "chronic condition". Chronic conditions are increasing with "multi-morbidity" (people with 2 or more chronic conditions) becoming the rule rather than the exception. Half of the over 75 have 2 or more chronic conditions, whilst 2 out of 75+ have four or more chronic conditions.[76] Mono-disease programs will not be able to address this problem. There will be a need for a paradigm shift from a disease-oriented care towards a care starting from the goals of the patient (see Chapter 3).[70] Primary Health Care will play an important role in avoiding fragmentation of care and enhancing integrated care. An increase in the number of vulnerable people will challenge the intensity and quality of interprofessional co-operation.
- **Scientific and technological** developments and their consequences for the affordability of care. Scientific progress offers a perspective of new preventive and curative opportunities in the field of genetics, cardiovascular diseases, neurosciences, cancer care and mental health. Information and communication technology form an integral part of daily practice. Hospital stay shortens continuously with an increase of day-hospitalisations (e.g. day-surgery), shifting more technological interventions to the home care. Primary care has a role to play in translating the new insights into practice with a focus on the "relevance" of the care, avoiding medicalisation of daily life[12] (see Chapter 5) . A lot of those new technologies and medications have an important impact on the budget of health care, requiring scientifically sound and socially accountable choices.
- **Socio-cultural** developments lead to the fact that the "patient" behaves more and more as a "consumer", presenting new questions related to

care to providers, based on information they found on the internet. Moreover, citizens are frequently invited for screening, check-up,… sometimes creating new worries (see Chapter 4). The changing societal context (more and more people work longer and claim for a better work-life balance) has an important impact on the availability of informal care (decreasing availability of volunteers, informal care givers,…). There is a clear change in the opinions about quality care at the end of life. The "existential" components of life as a human being become more and more important. Giving meaning to life is what matters for people. Patients want to give direction to their care starting from what they really value.

- In the **socio-economic** domain there are important health differences between countries, but also between social groups within the same country: "poverty causes illness, and illness causes poverty" is still reality. There is a clear widening social health gap in Belgium. A recent survey by the Scientific Institute For Public Health indicates that 47.2% of men with a low education level have a bad health condition, compared to 20.4% of men with higher education; men with a low educational level have chronic conditions twice as often as men with a higher education[197] (see Chapter 2). The financial and economic crisis has increased the social inequalities in health.[198] Today, 15% of the Belgian population lives below the poverty threshold, in the city of Brussels this is 33%.
- **Globalisation** leads to a more diverse and more multicultural care. People look at the international market in order to find solutions for their health problems. There is a concentration of people with different cultural backgrounds in cities, leading to the fact that "global problems" become more and more visible at the local level.

Reforming Primary Health Care in Flanders (Belgium)

The proposal the four professors formulated in "Together We Change" consisted of important structural changes at the micro, meso and macro level.

At the **macro level** a "Flemish Institute for Primary Care" had to be established (as already proposed in 1983), coordinating the regional policy with the federal legislation (and trying to influence that legislation in order to re-orientate the policy towards strengthening primary care). Moreover, the "Flemish Institute" should co-ordinate with the structures that support the local authorities and with the expertise centres related to specific topics (disease prevention, sexual and reproductive health, addiction,...). Their direct action should go towards supporting the meso level in terms of innovation and quality assurance. Moreover, the "Flemish Institute" should act as a "back office" in order to fulfil all the administrative tasks that facilitate the work at the meso level (data collection, analysis, payments,...). The "Flemish Institute" should also advice the regional government on formulating appropriate "health goals" for the Flemish Community. At the **meso level** 60 to 65 "Primary Care Zones" could become operational, each of them taking care of a population between 75,000 and 125,000 inhabitants and geographically organised in a way that they respect the borders of the local villages and cities. One Primary Care Zone could be composed of different neighbouring local entities (villages or cities). The co-operating communities that build together a Primary Care Zone receive a "reference budget" based on the "needs" of their population. The governance of the "Primary Care Zone" is supervised by a "Health Council", that is partly composed with administrators active in the local communities, and partly with representatives of patients/citizens, representatives of providers in health and welfare and representatives of the insurance companies (sickness funds).

At the **micro level** the supply is organised based on "Primary Care Networks", consisting of family practices, Community Health Centres, nursing services, social work, public welfare centres, pharmacists, physiotherapists, occupational therapists, nursing homes, organisations of informal care givers and volunteers, preventive services, home care services,... These Primary Care Networks are accountable for at least 10,000 people in urban areas and 5,000 in rural areas. The citizens are enrolled in a "Primary Care Network", through the fact that they subscribe to a patient list of one of the family medicine practices/community health centres belonging to that network. This organisational model guarantees that all inhabitants have access to a primary care network and are entitled to access all the services provided (nursing, social work, pharmacy,...) by the network. The citizens freely choose the primary care network. The Primary Care Network is responsible for a full accessibility for the citizens on its list and for sharing information, guidance and protocols and organising care continuity for its patients. Networks may co-operate at the level of Primary Care Zones within the framework of a Community-Oriented Primary Care approach in order to address the upstream causes of health problems (see box at the beginning of this chapter).

The Primary Care Zone is accountable for all the inhabitants in their geographical circumscription. In the future, a form of "vertical competition" can be organised between Primary Care Zones, so that, taking into account the differences in needs, Zones with better outcomes on relevant indicators can enjoy supplementary funding e.g. for investment in innovation.[199]

Primary Care Zones in Estonia

In a report entitled "Strengthening the Model of Primary Health Care in Estonia", commissioned by WHO Europe, the concrete strategy to implement a system of "Primary Care Zones" was described.[200] The report states: *"Organising primary care in decentralised entities, e.g. Primary Care Zones (PCZs), can contribute to the visibility of primary care. Defining the population who accesses a certain group of services and providers in primary care, can contribute to the accountability of providers in terms of outcomes, access and quality of care. A decentralised organisation of primary care can also create opportunities for co-operation with local authorities. This could contribute to better co-ordination between the health and social sectors. Moreover, a decentralised primary care can be used as a platform to attract and recruit candidates for training in health professional education programs, especially the recruitment for remote and rural areas. Decentralised PCZs may facilitate benchmarking and overall performance assessment"*. The report describes the functions of a Primary Care Zone (see box 4).

Box 4: Functions of the Primary Care Zone

- Provide support to the micro level by ensuring organisation and mentorship between different disciplines including family doctors and stimulating multidisciplinary and intersectoral co-operation, especially the most needed integration of health and social care.
- Organise continuity at the primary care level, for different disciplines (family medicine, pharmacy, nursing,...). This population-oriented continuity is different from the patient-related continuity of (planned) care at the micro level: the practice.
- Implement national programmes for health promotion, disease prevention, curative services, care and rehabilitation, in an integrated manner in order to provide universal access to those programmes.
- Facilitate the co-ordination between primary, specialised and hospital care with particular emphasis on patients' transitions (referral and discharge).
- Implement the provision of human resources for health care (recruitment and retention).
- Interact with national health authorities in order to inform priority setting and eventually adaptation of national policies.
- Facilitate different forms of citizen participation.
- Prepare agreement on complementary health goals, relevant for the PCZ.
- Optimise the utilisation of resources at the PCZ level.
- Assess performance of the PCZs and compare to other PCZs (after controlling for differences in need).

It is obvious that such an important reorganisation requires a clear change management strategy to reconcile bottom-up aspirations of municipalities with top-down requirements in terms of equity, accessibility, relevance and quality. The ownership by all stakeholders of the transition process is of utmost importance.

Will Change Happen in Flanders?

In order to make the change happen, the creation of more integrated interprofessional practices will be necessary. Apart from the Community Health Centres that use the Integrated Needs-Based Mixed Capitation System (see Chapter 9) and have already a "patient list", there are more and more multidisciplinary group practices that facilitate the co-operation between disciplines. According to international comparisons, however, Belgium has still a long way to go in order to increase the supply of interprofessional primary care services. Especially the intersectoral co-operation between health and welfare is still in its infancy, but we also have to look at education and housing.

On 16 February 2017 the Flemish Primary Care Conference took place and agreed to establish a "Flemish Institute for Primary Care" and the organisation of primary care according to the concept of Primary Care Zones as described in this chapter. There is some hesitation to start with the concept of interprofessional Primary Care Networks, as some stakeholders think that this will restrict too much the "freedom of choice" of patients. But the fact that the Flemish Minister is committed to make the "Primary Care Zones" and the "Flemish Institute for Primary Care" a priority is a positive sign.

In the past 40 years continuous efforts to establish a strong primary care system have faced a lot of hurdles and opposition.

Opposition comes very often from hospitals, certainly in hospital-centric countries. But all countries have huge difficulties to cut their (acute) hospital beds. In a recent report the OECD (Organisation for Economic Co-operation and Development) documented that the average annual decrease of hospital beds between 2000 and 2014 was less than 2% in OECD-countries.[201] On the other hand more and more hospitals co-operate in networks and perceive their task as "supporting primary care" through an integrated approach.

Other resistance very often comes from private independent providers, certainly when they work in a fee-for-service system, because they have almost no incentive to engage in co-operation with other services and disciplines. Here there are also positive evolutions e.g. the increasing co-operation between family physicians, pharmacists and nurses in the framework of "pharmaceutical care".

From the population there is sometimes opposition based on the argument of "freedom of choice". Of course, higher educated patients are able to organise the care for themselves, even in complex situations because they have the information needed and the financial and social capital to contact the providers they need. However, at the population level there are a lot of people who have neither the resources nor the "social capital" to take that responsibility themselves, and so organising accessible care teams who are used to work together is more equitable. Moreover, the scientific evidence points in the direction that "Teams are more effective than single practitioners in providing a range of important outcomes for the organisations, for the team members and for the patients".[202] There is evidence that teams with a fixed composition that are more diverse and work together for a longer period, lead to more effectivity and patient-oriented care. When looking at patients with chronic conditions, teams with a "fixed composition" see that their patients stay for a longer period of time at home, compared to control groups with "usual care" and "loose teams".

Health Policy Between Ideology and Evidence

Policy decisions are very often not based on "evidence", but on "ideology". Nowadays, in a lot of countries, politicians try to demonstrate that their ideology based on the principle that any problem will be resolved with a free market, should also be tested in health care, including primary care.

There is actually not a single experiment somewhere in the world that has demonstrated that the free market and commercialisation of health care is able to provide a health system based on relevance, equity, quality, person- and people-centredness, and sustainability. On the other hand, also systems with strong top-down organisational models, like the Semashko, formerly used in Central- and Eastern-Europe in Soviet times, are not able to address the challenges adequately. So, sustainable systems should be based on solidarity and social justice, should be person- and people-centred, sufficiently funded, bringing people to an adequate level of health literacy, and need providers that assure accessibility, quality, connectedness, commitment and accountability towards a population.

International Developments in Organisation of Family Medicine and Primary Care

After the publication of the World Health Report "Primary Health Care: Now More than Ever!" in 2008[203] the World Organisation of Family Doctors (WONCA), under the leadership of Professor M. Kidd (Flinders University, Australia), started to update its guidebook "The Contribution of Family Medicine to Improving Health Systems", leading to a second edition in 2013. This book clearly stressed the need for a "health system" approach, and the importance of accountability of family medicine towards a population.[204] The World Health Organisation emphasised in 2013 the importance of research for universal health coverage, in order to secure access to quality health services.[205] The important message of Chapter 3 of the WHR 2008 "Primary Care: putting people first" was operationalised in the WHO Global Strategy on People-Centred and Integrated Health Services, underpinned with a document "People-Centred and Integrated Health Services: an overview of the Evidence".[206] On 26 September 2015 the Bill & Melinda Gates Foundation, World Bank Group, and World Health Organisation launched a collaboration to strengthen primary health care and advance progress towards Sustainable Development Goals in New York: the "Primary Health Care Performance Initiative".[207] Dr Margaret Chan, director-general of the World Health Organisation said: "*Strong primary health care systems are where people turn in their communities to stay healthy and get care when they fall sick. When primary health care works, it can meet the vast majority of people's health needs.*" In the WHO-European Region (Copenhagen) a "European framework for action on integrated health services delivery" was developed, in order to inspire more integrated care, especially to address the challenges of chronic conditions and multi-morbidity.[208] Moreover, the WHO-Regional Office for Europe opened in Almaty (Kazakhstan) a WHO European

Centre for Primary Health Care. In June 2017 a first meeting of the "Primary Health Care Advisory Group", advising the Regional Director, convened in Almaty.

The European Commission selected an "Expert Panel on Effective Ways of Investing in Health" in order to advise the Commission in health matters. This Expert Panel also already focused on primary care issues in two of its "opinions": "Definition of a frame of reference in relation to primary care with a special emphasis on financing systems and referral systems" (2014) and "Tools and methodologies for assessing the performance of primary care" (2017). Since 2013 I am chairing the Expert Panel and enjoy a critical, constructive, open-mined co-operation of all the panel members.

In Europe the European Forum for Primary Care (www.euprimarycare.org) was the first organisation to formally bring the organisation of different health and welfare professionals in primary care together at European level.

The European Forum for Primary Care: Creating an Interprofessional Network

The European Forum for Primary Care (EFPC) was established in 2005. During the Dutch EU-presidency in the second half of 2004 a conference on the topic of "Competition in Health Care versus Social Accountability" was organised at which a group of driven family physicians and other primary care experts discussed the need for a broader scope on primary care. In the same period the Dutch Health Council issued the "European Primary Care" report recommending the establishment of a European Network for Primary Care. In existing international organisations the emphasis was on single professions and not on the broad range of primary care professions, policy-makers and researchers.

The launch of the EFPC took place in the premises of the European Parliament in Brussels, spring 2005, with a group of key representatives from different European professional groups. At this meeting I became the first chairman of the network with the support of D. Aarendonk, co-ordinator. The secretariat of the organisation soon moved to Nivel, The Netherlands Institute for Health Services Research in Utrecht, under patronage of Professor P. Groenewegen, Director of Nivel between 2009 and 2015.

From the onset the goal of EFPC was to create a sound, self-supporting network that finally became a legal entity in the form of an association, with registered members from autumn 2011 onwards. In April 2017 the association had approximately 100 institutional members and 65 individual members. EFPC managed to integrate almost all European organisations of all disciplines active in primary care and represented in the advisory board. On the 1st of October 2017, Prof. Sally Kendall, professor of Community Nursing and Public Health (University of Kent, UK), became the chair of EFPC.

When it comes to advocacy in the first years, EFPC got already a strong voice in supporting decisions that could contribute to the development of primary care: in 2009 at the World Health Assembly, EFPC, together with WONCA, supported the Resolution WHA62.12 "Primary health care, including health system strengthening".[209] More recently, at the World Health Assembly 2016, EFPC and WONCA managed to get a special side event with the World Federation of Public Health Associations (WFPHA) on the need for co-operation between public health and primary care.

At the crossroads of societal change, the experience of EFPC, illustrates that building worldwide co-operation between professionals from different disciplines active in primary care, including the social sector, is a key strategy to strengthen the primary care movement.

Reflection by Peter Groenewegen

The classical attitude of GPs used to be (and often still is) that if a patient does not call the doctor, s/he is apparently healthy. As this chapter shows, this attitude has to change as a result of demographic and epidemiological developments. More elderly people, people with chronic illness and handicapped people are living in their own homes longer. This is reinforced by policy changes with an eye to sustainability of long-term care.[210]

This asks for two developments. First of all outreaching primary care; the attitude should be: we are responsible for the people living here, whether they visit the practice or not. And secondly, it asks for involvement of the population with the primary care facility.

The outreaching attitude should be supported by appropriate organisation of practices and funding systems. Multidisciplinary practices with a community orientation is the organisational answer to the changing situation of care needs in the community. According to the QUALICOPC-study, in Europe there are still several countries with predominantly single-handed practices, among them Belgium, Austria, Germany, and countries with large multiprofessional teams, such as in Lithuania, Finland and Spain.[211] Although in the past, the Netherlands would have fitted in with the first group of countries, it is now above average in terms of different professionals in primary care teams. This is not so much the result of focused policy, but rather the by-product of the rules for reimbursement of practice nurses. In the same European study, GPs were asked three questions about their community orientation: whether they would report potential repeated accidents in an industry, frequent respiratory problems in patients living near a particular industry, and repeated cases of food poisoning among people living in a certain district. GPs in Norway, Turkey, Greece, Italy and the Netherlands most often say that they react to the described situations, whilst GPs in Cyprus, Estonia, Hungary, Germany and Latvia least.[212] In this respect, Belgium is at the lower half of the distribution. Both regarding practice organisation and community organisation, there is a lot to improve in Europe in general and in Belgium in particular.

The second required development is community and patient involvement at different levels. At micro level patients should be more engaged in their own health and care, e.g. through shared decision-making. At practice level members of the community should be engaged in running the primary care facilities. And at policy level patient organisations should be engaged in policy-making. Developments at these levels should be aligned to be able to reinforce each other. There is as yet no European comparative information about the state of patient and community involvement in primary care. The European Forum for Primary Care is developing a position paper on this subject.

Both required developments should not be independent. Multiprofessional organisation and community orientation of primary care and community and patient involvement should go hand in hand. The policy plans for the Flemish Community in Belgium, sketched in this chapter, have the potential to bring Belgium to a top primary care system.

Peter Groenewegen (1952) is a sociologist. He works as senior researcher at NIVEL and as endowed professor at Utrecht University. His research areas are primary care (in international perspective), sociology of the professions, and environment and health.

Chapter 9:

How to Pay Family Medicine and Primary Care?

In 1993 Goran joined the SERB Volunteer Guard with 4000 paramilitaries under the command of Arkan, to bolster the Republic of Serbian Krajina to fight against the Croatians in the Balkan war. During the fights in the region of Vukovar, Goran was wounded by a shrapnel, a grenade, full of metal bullets, that destroyed his left foot and the inferior part of his left leg. After first aid he received in Vukovar Hospital, he decided to flee to Western Europe as he could be of no use anymore in the war.

Some weeks later he arrives at the Community Health Centre Botermarkt and together with the nurse I do the inspection of his left leg and foot. The situation is disastrous: infected wounds, multiple metal bullets still present in the destroyed muscles and bones, an important infection. Goran was undocumented, so there was a problem to access hospital care and especially the needed surgical intervention. So we started systemic antibiotic therapy and local wound care in the primary care setting. The nurses took responsibility for the follow-up and in the meantime together with the social workers, we investigated the possibilities for a referral to a surgeon. The Public Centre For Social Welfare in the city of Ghent agreed to refund the surgical intervention, provided we could find a surgeon who could perform this for a "reasonable price".

After 3 weeks with visits to multiple surgeons, we found a surgeon who was willing to do the intervention for € 2500. The Public Centre for Social Welfare agreed, and intervention could take place. Our nursing team took care of the post-operative follow-up.

Later on the Royal Decree on "Urgent Medical Care" (12 December 1996) organised in a structural way the financing of "urgent care" for undocumented people. Family physicians can be reimbursed for this care in a fee-for-service scheme through the Public Centre for Social Welfare that receives the needed resources from the Federal Government. The system secures that there is no information from these transactions going to the Department of Home Affairs, responsible to deal with the legal situation of "undocumented people".

This story illustrates that before one can think about how to finance primary care, there is need for "Universal Health Coverage" and access to health care services, integrating all the people on the territory.

12 December 1997 at St-John's College, Cambridge (United Kingdom)

The prestigious buildings of St-John's College in Cambridge were the venue for a conference with 57 delegates representing 56 countries on the topic "Physician Funding and Health Care", organised by the Royal College of General Practitioners in conjunction with the World Health Organisation (WHO) and the World Organisation of Family Doctors (WONCA).

In preparation of this conference, the Department of Family Medicine and Primary Health Care of Ghent University was asked, together with the Netherlands Institute of Primary Care (NIVEL), represented by Professor Peter Groenewegen, to prepare a literature review on payment systems.[213] The review concluded: "Our analysis suggests that a capitation-based system of payment should most appropriately form the basis of any system of physician payment. In addition to this financial mainstay a combination of the other payment systems will be required to finance most appropriately the work of family physicians and their professional colleagues. The most suitable combination will depend upon the budget available and the particular country in question. The complexity and variety of tasks undertaken by a family physician working in primary care are considerable and require a similarly flexible and innovative system of physician payment". The review described in detail the effects of different payment systems on provider, patient and society, (fee-for-service, capitation, integrated capitation, salary) and documented essential conditions for the different systems in order to achieve their goals.

After long debates that took into account historical and geographical differences between primary care systems, the conference could agree upon a set of recommendations, including amongst others:

- Governments (national, regional,...) and state should be responsible for ensuring that all citizens are included in a health system which provides appropriate cover across a broad range of essential health services.
- The co-ordinating role of the family physician across the continuum of health care provision is highly cost-effective from the point of view

Family Medicine and Primary Care

of both individual patients and the health care system, and this activity should be promoted.

- The registering of individual patients (patient lists) with a given physician or practice is of great value to practices and health care planners in organising and administering services effectively and in determining accountability for the services provided. The essential range of health services to be provided within the health care system should be agreed by involving patients and communities in setting priorities. The provision of services to specific individuals should be determined by their primary care team in accordance with that person's clinical need, goals, preferences and the care available (see Chapter 3).

- All medical and health care students should study health economics in order to be educated about the issues involved in the allocation of resources.

- No single form of payment system can appropriately remunerate the complexity of tasks carried out by a skilled and trained family physician and a primary care team. An appropriate system of funding of physicians and other primary care team members is based on a mixed payment system which combines a number of the following: basic funding, capitation fees, weighted capitation payments, fees-for-services, target payments and sessional payments. Physician and primary care team funding policies should be value-led and encourage the implementation of a primary care-led health system which should aim to serve the entire population.

- There should be equity of remuneration between generalists and specialists. Both generalists and specialists are dealing with complexity: the generalists with the diagnostic complexity of early non-specific symptoms and complaints, often presented in the framework of a complex context (psycho-social determinants, cultural determinants,...), the specialists mainly dealing with technical complexity.

In this list the conclusions of the conference, that were focusing on physician funding, have been broadened towards the perspective of the interprofessional primary care team.

The following paragraphs describe my personal journey through different payment systems in primary care between 1978 and 2017.

1978: Starting in Fee-for-Service

When we started our practice in Ledeberg, the fee-for-service was the only operational payment system at the primary care level. The patient paid at the end of the consultation the full fee of the services provided and then sent his invoice to the Insurance Company that reimbursed 66% to 75% of the cost to the patient. For a small group of low income people (family income less than € 15,000 per year) this reimbursement could increase to 90% of the cost.

A "nomenclature list" documented the different types of provider-patient encounters that could be reimbursed (consultation in the practice, home visits, night visits, weekend visits,...) and defined between one hundred and two hundred items that could be additionally charged to the patient with a specific reimbursement (some blood tests, some interventions like putting stitches, interpreting electrocardiographic examination, cryotherapy for warts,...).

One major disadvantage of the system is that patients have to pay out-of-the pocket at the moment of the provider-patient encounter. Of course there was a "Third Party Payment"-system where the patient only had to pay his/her co-payment and the remaining part of the fee was paid directly by the insurer to the provider, but certainly in pre-computerised times, this was a very cumbersome and lengthy procedure. Undoubtedly, the system had a negative impact on accessibility of family practice and primary care, especially for poor people, who frequently chose to access an emergency department directly, where there was no need for direct payment and the invoice only arrived months later.

A difficulty in fee-for-service is also that, certainly in primary care, when the family physician – seeing e.g. a child with undefined symptoms like fever, cough,... – in the framework of good quality care proposes a follow-up visit in the forthcoming 24 hours, this will include that the patient has to pay a second visit. So, fee-for-service hinders both diagnostic and therapeutic continuity and follow-up. A third problem with fee-for-service, is that it limits possibilities for task-shifting and competency sharing: as family physicians and primary care nurses both have their own separated nomenclature, a physician who wants to shift some tasks to a nurse, will see his own income decrease, whilst the nurse's income increases. This is not really a base for "horizontal integration". A fourth disadvantage is that when using a "call-recall" system in the framework of prevention and screening the fact that the patient will have to pay for this encounter can reduce the accessibility of preventive care. A fee-for-service system, based on payment of defined interventions does not stimulate an integrated approach, as is needed in patients with multi-morbidity. Another challenge under the typical fee-for-service model is that there is continuous pressure, because doctors are incentivised to see more patients for less time to maximise profits. Finally, a nomenclature list of technical interventions will stimulate that physicians focus on the reimbursed interventions that are integrated in the nomenclature list, but will not perform other interventions, e.g. they will perform cryotherapy, but not counselling on healthy food.

In summary, fee-for-service is appropriate for short-term reactive care (e.g. somebody cuts his finger and the family physician puts the stitches and the problem is fixed), but it does not stimulate prevention and comprehensive integrated care, and does not contribute to accountability and equity from the societal perspective.

In the interprofessional team of the Community Health Centre we looked for a system that could overcome some of the limitations of fee-for-service.

1982: the Birth of Capitation; 1995: the Implementation

From international literature and from experiences in countries like Denmark, the Netherlands,... our Community Health Centre became informed about possibilities for payment in primary care based on a capitation system. We immediately saw the opportunities, but also the challenges: in the countries with a capitation system patients were "on a practice list", and could easily be identified. In the fee-for-service system in Belgium, this was not the case.

In 1981, after studying the Belgian legislation, we came across the fact that historically, when the Belgian social security system was established according to a Bismarck-approach, where social security was paid predominantly based on contributions by employers and employees in the framework of the social organisation of the country, the government was envisaging 3 types of payment: the completely liberal system, where doctors could ask what they wanted for the services they delivered to patients, the system based on "agreements" between health insurance and providers, where providers committed themselves to respect the tariffs that were agreed upon in the framework of the fee-for-service system and the patients would have the right to defined levels of reimbursement for every single service, and a third system which should be based on a "lump sum" financing, but that was never specified in the legislation. This third system was described in article 34 of the law on the "Health and Disability Insurance".

Two representatives of Community Health Centres of the French-speaking part of Belgium and Dr Ri De Ridder and myself, representatives of Community Health Centres in the Dutch-speaking part, had written a letter to request the implementation of the legislation in the framework of (interprofessional) primary care.

From the very beginning of the negotiations it was clear that the new system could only be accepted when it did not increase the expenses for primary care services, so the average expense for patients in the fee-for-service system and in the new system should be equal. This point was very much emphasised by the representatives of the insurance companies in the National Institute for Health and Disability Insurance (NIHDI).

During the process the Commission came across some very interesting data. In some of the provinces, e.g. East Flanders (capital: Ghent), the average spending for e.g. family medicine was twice as much as in the province of Brabant (capital: Brussels): 1.200 francs per year versus 600 francs per year. The reason was quite obvious: in the absence of a gatekeeping system and with an oversupply of hospitals and specialist services in Brussels the expenses were lower for primary care, but much higher for secondary care. This finding illustrated an important fact when it comes to taking decisions about financing systems: those decisions cannot be taken at the primary care level without debating the establishment of a gatekeeping system to secondary care. Another important challenge was that the insurance companies were not able to identify expenses at the level of an individual: expenses mostly were bundled at the level of a family. As the patients in the capitation system had to subscribe to a practice at the individual level, the monitoring of the system became a difficult challenge.

One of the important issues in the debate was whether or not there would be a cost-sharing ("co-payment") by the patients in the capitation system. The principle the Community Health Centres defended was that there is no reason to restrict the access of the population to the most cost-effective level of care (being the primary care). So, the agreement was that no co-payment by the patient was required. Another reason why Community Health Centres did not want a co-payment is that they were mostly working in deprived areas, with people for whom a co-payment would mean refraining them from access to primary care.[142] However, a consequence was that the average income of a family doctor in the capitated system would be 25 to 33% less than in the fee-for-service system.

Finally, it was important that the agreement was negotiated not only for family physicians, but also for nurses and physiotherapists. This was a strategy put in place by the Community Health Centres, as they wanted the payment system to support their interprofessional co-operation in primary care teams. Although Community Health Centres sometimes also included social workers and psychologists, these disciplines could not be integrated as there was no correlate in the fee-for-service system for the payment of these disciplines.

At the end of 1 year of negotiations the final agreement was approved in July 1982 and from the perspective of the Community Health Centres we were positive about important achievements: the fact that the agreement integrated 3 disciplines, the fact that the national solidarity was maintained, enabling also practices to start in places with a weak primary care system (e.g. Brussels); the fact that there was no co-payment for the patient and that the system was built on a patient list principle. Of course, when looking from an international perspective, it was a little bit strange that in Belgium Community Health Centres had to negotiate for a year in order to achieve what was already settled since 1949 in countries like Denmark and the Netherlands.

The implementation was a slow and time-consuming process, not in the least because everything had to be organised on paper (there was almost no computerisation in the health insurance companies). In the French-speaking part of Belgium the regional minister supported the start-up of Community

Health Centres with considerable seed money (4 million francs or € 100,000), enabling the French-speaking Community Health Centres to take momentum.

At the Flemish side there was no support at all from the regional government, so it took until 1993 before the first Community Health Centre started in the capitation system and the Community Health Centre "Botermarkt" was the second to switch in 1995.

One of the weak points of the capitation system was that it was completely linked to the expenses in the fee-for-service system. Paradoxically, the more "overproduction" there was in the fee-for-service, the more resources were available in the capitated system. But e.g. when the reimbursement for consultations in the fee-for-service system decreased, due to an increase of the co-payment, the resources in the capitated system decreased as well.

In the nineties it became clear that centres functioning in the capitated system developed another type of health care than those in the fee-for-service system. A comparison of the population who had access to the capitated Community Health Centres with the population in the fee-for-service system, indicated clearly that the capitated system was much more accessible than the fee-for-service system. A study by the Federal Knowledge Centre "Health Care" in 2008 confirmed this finding. When the researchers tried to compare 27,000 patients in the capitated system with a "comparative sample" in the fee-for-service system, they found it impossible to find a comparative sample of 27,000 people in the fee-for-service system that was as deprived as the sample from the capitation system in the Community Health Centres.[214]

In 1991 the Commission on capitated primary care payments decided to increase the capitation fee with 10% in order to compensate for the higher workload that resulted from dealing with a more deprived population. A second assessment, looking at the use of medical imaging, laboratory testing, and the number of patients that were hospitalised, revealed that Community Health Centres in the capitated system used less medical imaging and less laboratory testing, compared to the average use in the fee-for-service system. It also revealed that less patients from the capitated system were hospitalised. This resulted in a second increase with 10% of the capitation fee. Finally, in 1997, a third adaptation to the calculation of the system was made, because there was evidence that 10% of the Belgian population never had contact with

Family Medicine and Primary Care

the primary health care system (because they were in prison, or because they systematically used specialist care,...). So, the denominator was decreased with 10%, leading to a global increase of the capitation fee between 1990 and 1997 with 31%. This was all negotiated in the Commission that dealt with the capitation agreements, composed of 50% with representatives of insurance companies, 50% with representatives of the capitated Community Health Centres.

The Rise of the Capitation System: from Scientific and Societal Support towards Political Disapproval

In the 21st century the number of capitated Community Health Centres increased steadily till 170 health centres in 2017, taking care of 3.5% of the Belgian population. Nowadays, all the Belgian provinces have Community Health Centres and some cities, like Ghent, have already 10 CHCs, taking care of 15% of the population.

The study by the federal Knowledge Centre Health Care, already mentioned, indicated, apart from the excellent accessibility especially for deprived people, also a level of quality that was at least as good as in the fee-for-service system and where differences appeared, the quality was better in the CHCs. It became clear that there was less antibiotic prescription in the Community Health Centres, and within the antibiotic prescription less broad spectrum antibiotics. There was also more rational use of diagnostic interventions. Patients in the Community Health Centre used fewer resources in ambulatory secondary care, indicating that the package of services delivered in primary care was more extensive than in the fee-for-service. For the health care system there was no difference in total cost for primary and secondary ambulatory care and for the patient the system was by far less costly (less co-payments).

The societal support for Community Health Centres was increasing: civil society organisations, health insurance companies, trade unions, patient organisations,... supported the development of Community Health Centres.

However, in 2016 the new Minister of Health from the neoliberal party decided to decrease the resources for the Community Health Centres with 11 million euros, in the framework of the austerity policy of the government. Moreover, the minister set up a "moratorium" putting an end to the recognition of new Community Health Centres in the country. The arguments of the minister were that the sector was increasing with 10% every year, but she "forgot" to mention that the expenses in the fee-for-service system decreased at least with the same amount, as those patients switched to the capitation system. This development illustrated once more the risk of health care being subject to "ideological profiling" by neoliberal right wing political parties. At the moment where international organisations like the World Health Organisation, but also the World Bank, emphasised the need for integrated person- and people-centred primary health care (see Chapter 8), and when there is increasing scientific evidence that integrated payment systems enhance the quality of primary care teams, and at a moment of increasing evidence that abolishing out-of-pocket payments facilitates the access to primary health care, especially for the most vulnerable groups,[215] this development illustrates how fragile innovative initiatives in primary care are when they are confronted with a minister who ignores scientific evidence and prefers short-term ideological profiling over serving the needs of the population. The most astonishing fact is that this minister of Health has been herself... a family physician.

From a "Flat Capitation" towards an "Integrated Needs-Based Capitation"

In 2010 there were indications that the capitated system had difficulties to survive. The main reason was that in the fee-for-service system family physicians changed their way of practising, replacing home visits (that in the nineties still represented 40% of the encounters) by "consultations" in the practice and reducing the number of encounters in the follow-up of chronic conditions. This led to a decrease in the resources spent per person in the fee-for-service primary health care, which had also an impact on the resources available in the capitation system (as both systems were linked). Therefore, the decision was made to make an "independent" budget available for the capitated system, and at the same time an approach was developed where the distribution of resources in the capitated system would be guided by the "needs" of the patients on the list in a certain CHC. A model was developed with 42 variables, describing the "need for care" of the population on the list. From 2013 onwards every year an "electronic picture" of the population on the list of a CHC has been taken, and then, using the set of 42 variables (age, gender, SES, morbidity, functional status,...), the "relative need" compared to the other centres of a CHC has been calculated. Although the actual approach has to be optimised (selecting better indicators that define more appropriately the care need at primary care level) an Integrated Needs-Based Capitation System is well-fit to respond to the demographical and epidemiological transition within the primary care system.

An Integrated Needs-Based Capitation System probably is the best system to pay interprofessional primary health care teams with a "patient list", because:

- it stimulates prevention, health promotion and self-reliance of the people;
- as there is a global payment for different disciplines, there is an incentive to task-shifting and subsidiarity between the disciplines involved;
- it prevents risk selection, as patients with a "high need" contribute to increase the "average amount per patient" for a certain CHC;
- it stimulates a global approach to a broad range of health problems, avoiding fragmentation.

Pay-for-Quality:
the Solution to All Problems?

The implementation of different ways of paying primary care physicians and attempts to improve quality of care, including the use of financial incentives to directly reward "performance" and "quality", is increasing in a number of countries. The Quality and Outcomes Framework (QOF) for family physicians in the UK is an example of a major system wide reform.

In 2011 a review by the Cochrane Library on "The effect of financial incentives on the quality of health care provided by primary care physicians"[216] concluded that "despite the popularity of these schemes, there is currently little rigorous evidence of their success in improving the quality of primary health care, or of whether such an approach is cost effective relative to other ways to improve the quality of care. There is insufficient evidence to support or not support the use of financial incentives to improve the quality of primary care. Implementation should proceed with caution and incentive schemes should be carefully designed and evaluated".

The UK's Quality and Outcomes Framework (QOF) is the world's largest pay-for-performance program. It was introduced for all family practices in 2004, linking up to 25% of family physicians' income to performance for more than one hundred publically reported quality indicators relating to management of chronic disease, organisation of care and patient experience.[217]

The previous studies that investigated pay-for-performance programs have noted that financial incentive schemes can lead to slight improvements in incentivised aspects of care, but other aspects might be negatively affected, and the effects on patient outcomes are variable. In one survey 75.9% of nurses reported feeling the framework was undermining the patient focus of the National Health Service.[218] The root cause of this is that QOF has put an agenda in the clinicians' heads that is not necessarily consistent with the patients' perceptions. As one exploration into the impact of the QOF concluded: "The QOF-scheme may have achieved its declared objectives of improving disease-specific processes of patient-care... but our findings suggest that it has changed... the nature of the practitioner-patient consultation".[219]

In July 2016 a first study on the impact of the introduction of the "Quality and Outcomes Framework" on mortality was published.[220] The primary outcome indicator was the mortality for those conditions that receive special attention in the QOF (ischemic heart disease, hypertension, stroke including transient ischemic attack, diabetes, chronic kidney disease, asthma and chronic obstructive pulmonary disease). The secondary outcomes that were assessed are: age-adjusted and sex-adjusted mortality for ischemic heart disease, cancer and all causes of death that were not included in the primary outcome. The study compares population data from the UK with data of a "synthetic" country based on data from countries without "pay-for-performance". Morbidity, composition of the population, socio-economic factors were modulated in a way that the "synthetic country" was comparable with the UK. The main conclusion was that, compared to the data from the countries where no pay-for-performance was introduced, there was no significant impact of the introduction of the QOF on mortality. So, the conclusion is that these major investments (5.86 billion pounds in total) did not lead to a significant reduction in mortality.

These findings should warn governments not to jump quickly into "pay-for-performance" or "pay-for-quality".

What Could Be a Reason for These Findings?

A hypothesis could be that pay-for-performance starts from a wrong assumption: care processes are not linear (stimulus-response) processes, but rather circular processes that to a large extent are characterised by complexity and where context plays an important role (see Chapter 6 and 7). Moreover, there is the risk that disease-oriented "pay-for-performance" initiatives may lead to the fact that "other conditions" receive less attention. This implies a risk of "inequity by disease": as a patient you better do not have the "wrong disease" (that is not integrated in the program).

Another finding is that pay-for-quality-programs show positive results in the short term (mainly at the level of process indicators), but these results are not sustainable. Moreover, the "epidemiological transition" with more and more people with chronic conditions and "multi-morbidity" leads to the fact that the implementation of disease-specific "guidelines" as "golden standards" becomes more and more problematic, because those guidelines are to a large extent based on scientific research where patients with multi-morbidity were excluded. In the United Kingdom there was an attempt to solve this problem by creating the opportunity for the family physician to "exclude patients" from the QOF-program. With increasing multi-morbidity this kind of exclusion risks to become very frequent. Moreover, addressing multi-morbidity requires a paradigm shift from disease-oriented towards Goal-Oriented Care, with the goals of the patient as a starting point for the care process (see Chapter 3). It is actually unclear how "Goal-Oriented Care" can be reconciled with pay-for-performance, because those goals are unique for every patient.

Conclusions in Relation to Payment of Primary Care Providers at the Crossroads of Societal Changes

- Nowadays, collecting social security contributions and taxes is under political pressure. However, it is obvious that a society with an increasing number of chronic conditions and multi-morbidity, with rising numbers of mental health problems,... probably in the future will have to spend between 8 and 12% or even more of its GDP to health care. Collecting money for health care requires a high level of solidarity and social accountability of a population. Indeed, in most of the countries we observe that on a yearly basis 30% of the resources are spent by 90% of the population, whereas 10% of the population spends 70% of the resources. Moreover, a large part of those 10% will die in that same year. So, it is a remarkable indicator of solidarity that a lot of societies are still able to commit their population to this effort. But nowadays, in many countries this solidarity is under pressure...

- There is a need for investment of more resources in primary care. With the shift of care from hospitals towards the community the "money has to follow the care". Apparently, in most of the countries this is a real challenge. Tessa van Loenen et al. made a systematic review on which characteristics of primary care organisation influence avoidable hospitalisation for chronic ambulatory care sensitive conditions. The findings suggest that through strengthening primary care by increasing the primary care physician supply and enhancing long-term relations between primary care physicians and patients, potentially avoidable hospitalisations will actually be avoided. This appeared to be even more important than how the actual primary care delivery is organised.[221] When looking at the impact of primary care organisation on avoidable hospital admissions for diabetes in 23 countries, the researchers found that there was no association between disease management programs and rates of diabetes-related hospitalisation. However, an important finding was that the higher the number of hospital beds in a country, the higher the number of avoidable hospital admissions. A country's number of hospital beds seems to have more impact than aspects of good primary care; or rather the effect of primary care in reducing avoidable admission appeared to be counteracted by hospital bed supply.[222]

- In the debate about shifting the resources from hospital care to primary care, the solution cannot be found in only strengthening the primary care system towards a system which is continuous and has adequate accessibility. Reducing avoidable secondary care use requires to look at the balance between primary care and secondary care supply instead of seeking the solution in primary care solely. Lowering the number of hospital beds may be an important driver in the process of reducing avoidable secondary care use.

- There is now evidence that provider continuity in family medicine makes a difference in total health care costs.[223] Patients who were visiting the same family physician had a lower cost for medical care. So, a patient list system linking people to a provider or a practice is a good idea.

- A study in 11 European countries found lower inequality in specialist utilisation among groups with a different level of education, in gatekeeping countries. This provides support for the benefits of regulating access to specialist care through gatekeeping.[224] It restricts inappropriate utilisation and increases equity.

- In a gatekeeping system 2 types of referral processes can be distinguished (see figure 3). There is the "linear referral process", meaning that a patient is transferred from one provider to another for a more specialised work-up. This linear model is most appropriate for people with new (non-life-threatening) health problems that may be unclear for patient and provider and therefore are best presented first at the primary care level. Usually, only around 10% of these problems will require linear referral to other providers. The second type is the "spiral" model of referral: for people with chronic conditions and especially for those with multiple conditions this may be the most appropriate type of referral. Patients are referred within primary care and between different levels of the system on an ongoing basis. This requires a high degree of co-ordination. Appropriate mechanisms should be put in place to optimise the gatekeeping process according to the different contexts.[225]

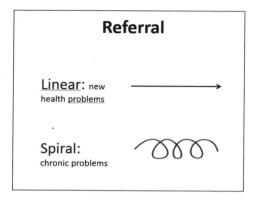

Figure 3. Two types of referral

- Efficient regulation of health care utilisation should take providers as its starting point and avoid regulations based on financial incentives such as cost-sharing for patients. Cost-sharing has been criticised in two ways. On the one hand, it has been argued that patients are not capable of deciding whether care is necessary at a certain point.[226] This argument is supported by empirical evidence that demonstrates that co-payments reduce both appropriate and inappropriate care. On the other hand, there are concerns about detrimental effects for the poor, who cannot afford the co-payments, even when care is necessary.[227]
- In a recent report the OECD (Organisation for Economic Co-operation and Development) summarises experiences of 12 countries, showing 3 broad recent trends in payment innovations:[228]
  - **add-on payments** paid on top of existing payment methods, which are tightened to specific expectations of the care provider. Such payments are being used to encourage co-ordination, improve care quality and reward performance;
  - **bundled payments** for episodes of care or for chronic conditions, which aim to improve care quality and reduce costs;
  - **population-based payments**, in which groups of health providers receive payments on the basis of the population covered in order to provide most health care services for that population, with built-in quality and cost-containment requirements.

  For primary health care the third approach (population-based payments, in which groups of health providers receive payments based on the population covered) is the best option. A blended payment scheme with a yearly risk-adjusted population-based global payment as basis,[229] eventually supplemented by pay-for-co-ordination and other quality-stimulating features, is most appropriate to answer the challenges from the epidemiological transition. Moreover, taking into account the importance of social determinants of health on the one hand and the increasing role of welfare in addressing chronic conditions and multi-morbidity on the other hand, a pooled budget to integrate health and social care may be an option.

- In health systems, where actually fee-for-service is the predominant payment system in primary care, a transition strategy will be needed. One of the possibilities is to systematically reduce the fee-for-service part and to increase the capitation-part.

- More knowledge is needed to optimise the indicators used in order to build an integrated needs-based capitation system. What are the important variables that contribute to the workload of a primary care team? This needs more practice-based research.

- There is actually no evidence to introduce "pay-for-performance" or "pay-for-quality" mechanisms in primary care. These linear stimulus-response mechanisms probably insufficiently grasp the complexity of primary care and the need for circular processes. If introduction of these mechanisms is debated, it is important to stress the need for appropriate information systems, documenting relevant process- and outcome-indicators, to limit the impact (5% of the income or less, paid at the level of the team) and to follow it up continuously, limiting the test period in time. There is a conceptual problem between "pay-for-performance" on the one hand and "Goal-Oriented Care" on the other hand.

Reflection by Lieven Annemans

If policy-makers want to take health seriously – and they should! – they know they have to make explicit choices about the organisation of the health care systems. Poor access to health leads to immense social losses. Mackenbach and colleagues calculated that in Europe inequity in health care is responsible for 20% of health care expenditure and for 700,000 deaths. But poor access is not only solved by making necessary care cheaper or even free. Good access also requires that there is a clear, visible and open gate for everyone. No one can be left behind. This means that every citizen should be mandatory registered at a primary care practice. Only then, care can be decently co-ordinated and exclusion can be avoided. How should the primary care practice then be paid? In this chapter Jan De Maeseneer argues correctly for a needs-based capitation system: a fee per month per registered patient. All physicians have a combination of intrinsic and extrinsic motivation in the conduct of their activities. Intrinsic motivation basically comes down to willing to help other people. Extrinsic motivation is related to the financial reward. It is thereby frustrating for physicians when they observe that those who practice badly in a fee-for-service system earn more money. In a capitation system this can be tackled since it involves an implicit pay-for-quality component: the better you care for your patients the more patients will be attracted to your practice. Obviously, the parameters that define the level of the per capita payment should be carefully selected. If there is too much focus on comorbidities this holds the risk that if patients are not well treated and get more complications then income for the physicians would increase because of the increasing number of comorbidities. A system which is more based on gender, age and especially socio-economic status would be more simple and fair. For physicians who currently work in a fee-for-service system a gradual increase in the fixed fee per registered patient would be the right track towards an integrated capitation system.

Finally, it becomes clear from this chapter that a primary care practice does not live on an island. On the one hand there is a need to reach out to the community and the environment of the patient, whereas on the other hand there is a need for frequent contact and communication with specialised care. This again requires a payment system that encourages these interactions.

Lieven Annemans, MSc, PhD, full professor of health economics at Ghent University, Faculty of Medicine and Health Sciences.
Member of the WHO Primary Health Care Advisory Group.
Previously chairman of the Flemish Health Council and advisor to the Minister of Social Affairs. Past-President of ISPOR (International Society of PharmacoEconomics and Outcomes Research).

Chapter 10:
Family Medicine and Primary Care in an International Context

A consultation that could have happened anywhere on earth.

This afternoon in 1997 I am observing consultations in the "Centro de Salud Chavez Rancho" in Cochabamba (Bolivia). A young family physician is taking care of patients.

A young woman enters the consultation room, complaining of a sore throat. There is no chair for the patient in the consultation room, and the doctor asks the patient to open her mouth, looks at the throat and prescribes antibiotics. Two minutes after she entered, she leaves the consultation room, but whilst opening the door and with the door handle still in her hand, she asks: "Doctor, tengo otra pregunta…" and before the doctor can intervene she starts telling about the difficult living conditions at home. She is a mother of 3 children, but increasingly, she suffers from intrafamily violence by her husband who is frequently beating her,… Recently, the children were involved in the violence and she is wondering what she should do. Her husband's alcohol abuse increases, and he lost his job.

The doctor listens carefully and reacts empathetically to the concerns, the fears and the hopelessness of the woman. He advises her to contact the social worker in order to be informed about her rights and the juridical procedures, and in any case when violence occurs, invites her to come immediately to the Health Centre.

We reflected together on what happened during this consultation. "How could I have known that there was also another agenda, apart from the biomedical one?", the family physician asks. We briefly discussed the importance of exploring the reason for encounter of any patient, even when the obvious complaint seems to be a quite simple medical question, as in this case. The question "Why does this patient come to see me now with this complaint?" could be helpful in guiding this exploration. As the Bolivian family physician asked for explicit feedback, I told him that he really has empathetic skills in his communication with patients. Before the next patient enters, he looks for a chair, so that a patient will no longer be standing during the consultation.

Although the context was specific, what happened in this consultation was universal and will be recognizable for everybody involved in primary care.

5 October 1995: Royal Automobile Club in London (Only for Men)

On 5 October 1995, following the suggestion by colleague Dr R. De Ridder (see Chapter 9), family physician in a Community Health Centre in Ghent, a meeting was arranged with Professor Dumo Baqwa (Primary Health Care, University of Cape Town, South-Africa) at the Royal Automobile Club in London (only for men). This location was chosen by one of the NGOs that was involved in supporting developmental work in South-Africa. Ri De Ridder had met with Professor Baqwa at a workshop in South-Africa on integrating interpreters and intercultural mediators in primary care and had informed me that the Professor was a very inspiring person.

The meeting was special, not only because of the location and environment, but because of the fact that, although we had never met before, we had similar ideas on many matters. Professor Baqwa explained the role he had played in the fight against Apartheid, working for the ANC (African National Congress), his exile to Europe and his training to become a physician in Germany, his commitment with Steve Biko in the long struggle against Apartheid, and how the death of Steve Biko influenced his life. As a student I had been involved in a lot of solidarity movements supporting the fight against Apartheid, but the person now in front of me, really did it. Dumo Baqwa explained that primary care was high on the agenda in South-Africa and that family medicine should be the medical discipline in the primary care team. He invited me for a study visit in order to meet the most important actors in the development of family medicine in South-Africa.

This trip to South-Africa was a "life-changing experience" for me: a visit to the townships in Crossroads and the Health Centre, visits to "informal housing" with a "family planning nurse" in Kayelitsha and listening to stories about rape and violence, meetings with Professor Sam Fehrsen (Medunsa), Professor Bruce Sparks (Witwatersrand), Professor Pierre de Villiers (Stellenbosch University),... In my conversations with all these heads of Departments of Family Medicine in the different universities, I shared our positive experience in Flanders with inter-university co-operation in the field of family medicine training (see Chapter 7). Most of the South-African heads of department were interested to explore the possibility of a co-operation between the Departments of Family Medicine in the 8 medical faculties in South-Africa.

The Family Medicine Educational Consortium

With a small financial grant from the Flemish Minister of Education a workshop was organised with the 4 Flemish departments and the 8 South-African departments, focusing on "Training in Family Medicine and Primary Health Care in South-Africa and Flanders", in September 1997 in Durban (South-Africa).[230]

After negotiations which were not always easy (in 1997 there were still huge racial differences in the composition of the different universities in South-Africa), all participants agreed and signed the "Durban Declaration", stating that *"The 8 departments responsible for family medicine in South-Africa agree to establish a Consortium for co-operation to reach common goals:*

- *establishing a network for communication and consultation;*
- *development of a common vision and co-operation for vocational training;*
- *looking for methods to disseminate the viewpoints of the consortium;*
- *the sharing and exchanging of expertise;*
- *the common use of resources, in order to develop service delivery, in all districts of the country;*
- *contribute to the necessary change strategy at the level of undergraduate training and vocational training for family medicine".*

Between 1997 and 2003 the FaMEC-Consortium (Family Medicine Educational Consortium) organised regularly inter-university meetings. One of the major challenges was the development of a common curriculum and the realisation of an appropriate evaluation system. From 2003 onwards the development had been financed by a project from the Flemish Interuniversity Council in order to contribute to the "Optimisation of the vocational medical training in family medicine/primary health care in South-Africa: a contribution to the realisation of health for all". The resources enabled the employment of a co-ordinator for the consortium (Professor Jannie Hugo, University of Pretoria) and a "Train the trainers" program was organised on a regular basis. Two groups of trainers from South-Africa had the opportunity to visit the Flemish Departments of Family Medicine, leading to an interesting exchange of experiences related to the didactics of training future family physicians. These interactions created a learning community with reciprocal North-South learning. Remarkably, there were huge similarities in strategy and educational developments, both in the North and in the South. In South-Africa, learning modules were developed in the framework of E-learning, the practical training was organised in "Training Complexes" (consisting of Primary Care Centres with the co-operating "clinics" and "District Health Hospitals"). In a short period of time 17 "Training Complexes" were developed in all provinces of South-Africa and students of different universities made use of the same "Training Complex".

Going East and North

The success of the developments in South-Africa was followed by contacts with starting Departments of Family Medicine and Primary Health Care in Tanzania, Uganda, Mozambique,... Based on the positive outcomes a new project was financed by the Belgian co-operation agency in 2006: "Development of training in family medicine/primary health care in Southern and Eastern Africa: a contribution to the realisation of quality and equitable health care through a South-South network". This project had 2 part-time co-ordinators: 1 for South-Africa and 1 for East-Africa. Apart from the 8 departments of South-Africa, the network included: Aga Khan University (Tanzania), Moi University (Eldoret – Kenya), University of Goma (DRC), National University of Rwanda (Kigali – Huye), Makerere University (Kampala) and Mbarara University of Science and Technology, both in Uganda. Following the principles of "South-South co-operation" the focus of the development of training programs was completely in the South. Strategies were developed in order to enable information-sharing, and this information was integrated in appropriate educational models, taking into account the different contexts and health systems in the participating countries. Handbooks, modules, training programs were exchanged and there was mutual participation with staff members acting as external examiners in each other's assessment of the students. In all the countries the model of "training complexes" was implemented as much as possible, with a special attention for social accountability (focusing on socially vulnerable groups).

Going North and West

From 2008 onwards the network got financing by the ACP-EU-Co-operation Programme in Higher Education (EDULINK) and was named: "Primafamed-network: Primary Care/Family Medicine Education Network".

The goals of that project were the following:

- a contribution to health of local communities, by a high quality health care delivery in sub-Saharan Africa through the training of family physicians working in the framework of an interdisciplinary primary care team, focusing on the needs of individuals and families and the community they live in;
- the development and strengthening of the training capacity of academic departments of family medicine, both in undergraduate and postgraduate training. The aim was to build a common vision and strategy, fit for purpose in sub-Saharan Africa, illustrating clearly the role of family medicine and primary health care, and building an institutional network between the departments of family medicine.
- apart from the 8 departments in South-Africa, other departments joined the network coming from Tanzania, Kenya, Uganda (2), Democratic Republic of Congo, Rwanda, Sudan, Ghana and Nigeria. The financial support by the European Union stimulated the start of new "Training Complexes" in the participating countries. Moreover, the project enabled "staff mobility" leading to the strengthening of local capacity for teaching and assessment.
- an important landmark in the development of the Primafamed-project was the launch of the *"African Journal for Primary Health Care and Family Medicine"* (www.phcfm.org) in 2008, with financing from Belgian development aid. This was probably the most cost-effective investment we ever made in developmental projects: the journal very quickly became a platform where the scientific research of family medicine and primary health care in Africa was documented. The launch took place at the first "Primafamed-workshop" in Kampala (Uganda), with the participation of more than one hundred stakeholders in family medicine and primary health care from the majority of the sub-Saharan countries. The African Journal was for many scholars the platform where they published their

first scientific paper and nowadays has become a self-sustaining project, with more than hundred articles published each year.

The research focused on exploring the basic principles of family medicine in Africa. Mash R et al. used a Delphi-consensus procedure in order to describe the basic principles.[231] This article illustrated clearly that the central values and characteristics of family medicine as holistic approach, longitudinal care, comprehensive approach and focus on family and local community were seen as important features, but with a different contextual specificity. There are also some specific differences with the situation in Western countries: almost no home visits by family physicians and the "practice population" that was mostly seen as the "district population". Moreover, certainly in rural and remote areas, where hospitals were not easy to reach, family physicians had to be able to perform certain procedures in surgery and obstetrics.

South-South Co-operation: the Twinning-Project

In June 2009 Primafamed received again funding by Belgian governmental aid for the project "Strengthening developmental capacity for family medicine training in Africa: the South-African family medicine-twinning project". In this project the principles of South-South co-operation became a strategy: each of the departments of family medicine in South-Africa started a "twinning" in order to train family physicians in countries and regions where there was no medical faculty, nor even a university. The role of E-learning programs in this project was central, and the establishment of local "training complexes" for the students was supported by the South-African "twinning departments". The "twinning entities" were University of Cape Town and University of Namibia (where on 1 February 2010 the cohort of the first year of the undergraduate medical curriculum started), University of Stellenbosch working together with University of Botswana (where a medical faculty just started in 2009), University of Orange Free State (Mangaung) co-operating with Lesotho, University of Witwatersrand (Johannesburg) twinning with Malawi (Blantyre), Walter Sisulu University (Umtata) twinning with Zimbabwe, University of Pretoria working with Swaziland and the Nelson Mandela University (Durban) co-operating with Mozambique. By developing these twinnings, "internal brain drain" within the African continent may be reduced: because previously there was a risk that students who were trained abroad (in the absence of a medical faculty in their own country) did not return to their country. This project has been evaluated as very positive and is still ongoing.

An important concern was the "Africanisation" of the Primafamed-network, also at the level of funding. Under the leadership of Professor Bob Mash the Department of Family Medicine and Primary Health Care of Stellenbosch University made a successful application for a grant from the European Union, for a project aiming at scaling up dramatically the number of physicians in primary care in South-Africa. This project also enabled international exchange in the framework of the Primafamed-network.

Scaling up of capacity increasingly became a focus of attention, certainly from a policy-makers' perspective. This concern was echoed by the "Statement of the Primafamed-network, Victoria Falls, Zimbabwe" in 2012 on "Scaling up family medicine and primary health care in Africa".[232] This document emphasises that, if the necessary conditions are fulfilled, it would be possible to train 30,000 new family physicians in the next 10 years. One of the strategies could be that 50% of the medical graduates should be trained in family medicine in order to contribute to the needed scaling up of capacity.

One of the inspiring programs for scaling up was the 2-year training program in family medicine in the community that was implemented by the faculty of medicine of Gezira University and the Ministry of Health in Sudan. This program addressed the needs of the local population, was supported by E-learning, and involved 207 candidates. The training program provided health services in 158 centres, of which 84 had never been served by a doctor before.[233]

Evaluation: a Difference Was Made

In the framework of the assessment of the EDULINK-project, Flinkenflögel M et al. described the change in developmental progress at the level of the participating departments. It became clear that all the departments made considerable progress both at the level of training and policy development in

2008-2011. The SWOT-analysis illustrated that support of the local departments is of utmost importance, especially support from the local authorities. Development of training of family physicians is possible, but it is a slow process. South-South co-operation is an effective strategy in order to strengthen family medicine development.[234] In the meantime there was also important and positive societal feedback towards the family medicine development. In the preface of the book by Hugo and Allen *Doctors for Tomorrow: Family Medicine in South-Africa* archbishop emeritus Desmond Tutu writes:

"Doctors in family medicine are aware of the challenges, attempt to understand them better and work to address them... The issues of principles and values, relationships and meaning are not left to chance, but become an important element of service, systems, training and research.

This gives me hope of a transformation in the health service that can take care of our people, which can guide us through this difficult time. This hope is not only for South-Africa, but also for our brothers and sisters in the rest of the continent and the rest of the world.

If the family medicine movement can play that role, let us join hands and realise that dream".[235]

From Research to Politics

In the framework of the EU-FP7 Research Program the Department of Family Medicine and Primary Health Care applied successfully with the project: "Human Resources for African Primary Health Care: HURAPRIM" (www.huraprim.ugent.be). The partners involved in this project were Ghent University, Oxford University (UK), Medical University of Vienna (Austria), Mbarara University of Science and Technology (Uganda), Aidenet NGO (Mali), Université de Bamako (Mali), Ahfad University for Women (Sudan), Witwatersrand University (South-Africa) and University of Botswana (Botswana). The project looked at the broader context of Human Resources for African Primary Care, including issues like training, brain drain,... Apart from the international brain drain, where health care workers leave to work in other continents, there is also a brain drain phenomenon within Africa.

Human resources are moving from rural areas to the cities, from primary care to specialty care, from the public services to private services, and from general health care to programs focusing on specific diseases such as HIV/AIDS. When looking at the graduates of one of the undergraduate medical training programs in the participating countries, HURAPRIM found that from the 790 trained medical doctors so far 88% were still working in the country, which was a very good result. However, 51% of the graduates were working for 1 single disease in the framework of an HIV-related non-governmental organisation, funded by external donors. This is a dramatic example of "internal brain drain", especially because a lot of those doctors actually fulfil administrative tasks in these vertical disease-oriented programs. From interviews with African doctors working abroad, it became clear that there are economic and political elements that determine the reason that people migrate: difficult work conditions, low salaries and very high workloads. Economic conditions are of course an important factor, but many people emigrate for other reasons, e.g. to specialise in a particular field, to escape political instability or insecurity, or to join family members who are already living abroad. These are understandable personal decisions, often taken in very difficult circumstances. Strategies to counter the phenomenon need to focus on structural solutions, that boost health workers' options at home. Addressing the problem is not simply a matter of money, although of course adequate financial resources are needed. Training health workers in their own country could already solve a part of the problem. Specific strategies to support family practice in underserved areas is needed. It is important that the medical graduates willing to work in remote rural locations could receive additional training and support over the internet, for example, enabling them to build up the required skills and autonomy.

HURAPRIM looked into the causes of brain drain, but also examined the consequences – for example by means of "virtual autopsies" of children deceased under the age of 5. The researchers interviewed the families and health workers involved in a number of cases and concluded that most of these tragedies could have been prevented. Where primary health care is unavailable or under-skilled, lives are lost. But there is also a responsibility "in the West". The international community should agree that if you integrate a doctor or a nurse who was trained in a developing country in your health system in the West, you should reimburse the full cost of training that person to the country of origin. This approach would enable countries of origin to train several people for every person that left.[236]

Researchers in HURAPRIM did not limit their actions to "observation". One of the observations was the very low monthly salaries of primary health care professionals in Uganda. When a debate took place in the Parliament as a consequence of the fact that the Minister had reduced the health budget considerably, the team from Oxford University and the University of Mbarara produced a document: "Why Uganda Needs to Increase its Health Budget: a Briefing for Members of Parliament", documenting the negative impact such a decision could have on maternal and child mortality. After the following debate the government announced that it would double monthly pay for doctors in health centres, and investment would be made to recruit 6.172 additional health workers.

This kind of approach linking evidence to action was also the reason why already in 2008 different organisations – WONCA (World Organisation of Family Doctors), GHETS (Global Health through Education, Training and Service), The Network: Towards Unity for Health and the European Forum for Primary Care (EFPC) – published an editorial in the *British Medical Journal*, asking donors of vertical disease-oriented projects to invest 15% of the budgets for vertical programs in strengthening co-ordinated and integrated primary health care. The organisations set up the 15by2015-campaign, calling for major international donors to assign 15% of their vertical budgets by 2015 to strengthening horizontal primary health care systems so that all diseases can be prevented and treated in a systematic way. The example of Mozambique illustrates the approach: in 2005 the total health expenditure in the country was $356m. Foreign assistance accounted for $243m, from which $130m was channelled through disease-specific vertical funds managed directly by donors. With 15% of that money 65 health centres could be supported for a year, with appropriately trained staff. This could give more than one million people access to improved primary health care.[6]

Going Global to Other Continents

Apart from its involvement in Africa with the Primafamed-network the Ghent Department of Family Medicine has also been active in Latin-America (Nicaragua, Ecuador, Bolivia) and in Asia (Vietnam, Thailand, China), trying to spread the training of primary health care providers, especially family physicians, worldwide. This co-operation had first of all a capacity-building component, in order to give more people access to quality primary health care. Moreover, there was a research component analysing the underlying "upstream causes" of the maldistribution of healthcare workforce worldwide. Finally, this co-operation also created an opportunity for the organisation of clerkships for our students "overseas". Nowadays, more than 1 out of 3 students work in one of the countries outside Europe for 2 to 3 months during his/her clerkship.

What did we learn from international co-operation?

Working for 20 years at the global scale, gave us the opportunity to interact with the best of "many worlds". We learnt from the enthusiasm, the idealism, the creativity of people in Africa, Latin-America, Asia. We understood that there is no need to "teach" Africans in "doctor-patient communication" and "empathy": their person-centred approach includes so many aspects of culture, interrelated connectedness, imagination,… that it was always a learning experience for us to assist in doctor-patient interactions. Participation of people in the health system was obvious in Latin-American countries with "local organisations operating at the level of the community: Organizaciones Territoriales de Base". We looked with an open mind at integration of Traditional Chinese Medicine with western "evidence based" approaches in health centres in China in order to re-construct the trust of the population in the health care system.

Whatever the context, the history or the culture, family medicine and primary care was recognised as the point of entry and the hub in the health system because of its continuity, comprehensiveness, person- and people-centredness. These core values of family medicine and primary care find their ways in multiform organisational patterns, trying to answer local needs (e.g. in rural and remote areas, where obstetrical and surgical skills are required at the primary care level).

The challenges are common: scaling up capacity, improving access and quality, and contribute to social cohesion.

Family medicine as a discipline is also a strategy against "brain drain", because the people who are able to perform best in primary care, are those who originate from the communities they are serving.

Another commonality with what happens in the western world is the need to invest more in primary care in order to enable the strengthening of health systems.

But, what I learned most: a deep respect for the optimism, the commitment, the solidarity of the people who continue to care for individuals and communities, especially those most in need, every day,... The moment I felt most honoured as an academic was when Dr Olayinka Ayankogbe, Senior Lecturer in Family Medicine and Head, Family Medicine Unit, Department of Community Health and Primary Care, College of Medicine, University of Lagos (Nigeria), gave me this feedback: "You are a black man in a white skin!".

Why This International Commitment? On a Personal Note...

Reflecting on what inspired me to engage in international co-operation, especially in Africa, of course the experience together with my wife Anita in Rwanda (see Chapter 1) in 1977 played an important role: once you are influenced by this mixture of challenges, problems, difficulties on the one hand and joy, hope, perspective and enthusiasm on the other hand, it is difficult not to return to Africa. But for me, I discovered that probably there is also another reason. My younger brother Paul (see Chapter 7) was a journalist to cover international news in Asia, Africa, and Latin-America for the Belgian Dutch-speaking broadcasting corporation. Unfortunately, he died on 18 May 1992 in Hong Kong. I always listened to his contributions on the radio from different places on earth. After his death, we wrote a book with colleagues and friends: *A Voice for the Third World*, because that was what he has always been. One way or another I felt that his job was not finished, and that I had to continue, contributing to give the developing world not only a voice, but also access to better primary care. By the way, as Paul wrote in one of his articles in 1985, was I not born in the year of the discovery of the "Third World", 1952?

The French demographist Alfred Sauvy wrote on 14 August 1952 an editorial in *France Observateur*: "Nowadays we talk a lot about the 2 worlds of the 'big powers', but we forget that there is also a 'third power', the most important one and in fact the first one that existed" and he finished: "Ce Tiers-Monde ignoré, exploité, méprisé, comme le Tiers-État, veut lui-aussi être quelque chose" ("this Third-World, unknown, exploited, despised, as the Third Estate, also wants to be something"). Sauvy chose the "Third World" in analogy with the "Third Estate", hoping that, just as the Third Estate made the French Revolution, the Third World could play a revolutionary role at global level too.

My brother Paul was a visionary person, who looked at the "global world" long before the term existed. At a lecture on the need for "societal education" in schools he concluded:

"The answer to the question whether or not our future will be worthwhile, will depend on the fact whether or not we choose for a life in integrity, and not a life in consumption; whether or not we will be able to create a way of life enabling us to be spontaneous and independent but connected to each other, instead of maintaining a way of life that only enables us to produce and to destroy, to produce and to consume, a way of life that is just a station on our way to exhaustion and pollution of the environment. This is not an easy choice". His words on 1 February 1980, at the age of 26.[237]

Reflection by Akye Essuman

Kampala, Uganda, September 2007. It was my first exposure to an international academic workshop. Hopefully, I would be able to present my work after observing some seasoned experts do theirs and pick up a few "tricks" of the trade... or so I thought. Then comes in this energetic workshop promoter who after the initial pleasantries announces... "Okay everybody, it's time to get down to business; we shall first listen to... Ghana!" Goodness, I felt like being pushed off the deep end and wished the ground would open and simply swallow me up. How I went through that presentation, which by the way was well received, now belongs to history.

I had joined the medical school in the University of Ghana earlier in 2007, two years after completing specialty training in family medicine through the West African programme. Together with another colleague, my mandate was to develop undergraduate family medicine. As the pioneer graduate, I was the local "expert". However, without an academic mentor in the specialty, the terrain became quite frustrating. That September, the dean, Professor Aaron Lawson, asked me to represent him at the Kampala workshop which he believed would be more beneficial to me (he was an anatomist). This workshop, which gave birth to the Primafamed Network project, proved to be a defining moment in my career as a family physician and the development of family medicine in Ghana. It became our gateway to global family medicine. Suddenly, I had access to experts in the specialty all over the world who provided mentorship in various aspects – curriculum development, teaching skills, presentation skills, research and publication etc. Primafamed provided opportunities to attend annual workshops and conferences, purchase textbooks (I had only two outdated editions), access journals and participate in the "staff mobility" programme.

Family medicine today in Ghana is a force to reckon with. The Ghana Health Service envisages to place at least two family physicians in all district hospitals in the shortest possible time. Training has been decentralised to the district training complexes instead of teaching hospitals.

It is the passion of most emerging academics from developing countries to have part of their training in institutions in developed countries. In most situations this results in brain drain. It is my firm believe that a means to curb the brain drain from Africa is to provide such opportunities as did Primafamed. Well structured, mutually respecting international collaborations promoted by persons with not only "gifted hands", but also "gifted hearts" and "gifted minds" will produce contented local experts with global relevance.

Akye Essuman, Lecturer and Acting Head, Family Medicine Unit, Department of Community Health, University of Ghana. Consultant Family Physician, Korle-Bu Teaching Hospital. Former Secretary and Training Co-ordinator, and current Chief Examiner, Faculty of Family Medicine, Ghana College of Physicians and Surgeons. Country co-ordinator, Primafamed Education Network.

Family Medicine and Primary Health Care at the Crossroads of Societal Change

In the 10 chapters of this book we looked at topics in relation to family medicine and primary care that underwent important changes in the last four decades. During 40 years I had the privilege to be part of these developments as a practising family physician, as an academic researcher, as a teacher and as someone involved in advising policy decisions in health care at different levels. I am extremely grateful for all the opportunities that I received from so many people.

Looking at the future is an important challenge today. In the past years society has changed a lot, and family medicine and primary care will have to participate in responding to the new contexts.

Pankaj Mishra, in a contribution to *The Guardian* on 8 December 2016, describes the changes and challenges:[238]

"We cannot understand this crisis because our dominant intellectual concepts and categories seem unable to process an explosion of uncontrolled forces.

In the hopeful years that followed the fall of the Berlin Wall in 1989, the universal triumph of liberal capitalism and democracy seemed assured; free markets and human rights would spread around the world and lift billions from poverty and oppression. In many ways, this dream has come true: we live in a vast, homogeneous global market, which is more literate, interconnected and prosperous than at any other time in history.

And yet we find ourselves in an age of anger, with authoritarian leaders manipulating the cynicism and discontent of furious majorities. What used to be called 'Muslim rage', and identified with mobs of brown-skinned men with bushy beards, is suddenly manifest globally, among saffron-robed Buddhist ethnic-cleansers in Myanmar,[239] as well as blond white nationalists in Germany. Violent hate crimes have blighted even the oldest of parliamentary democracies, with the murder of the MP Jo Cox[240] by a British neo-Nazi during the venomous campaign for Brexit. Suddenly, as the liberal thinker Michael Ignatieff recently wrote: "Enlightenment humanism and rationalism" can no longer adequately "explain the world we're living in."

Today, the human norm is the Homo economicus, a calculating subject whose natural desires and instincts are shaped by their ultimate motivation: to pursue happiness and avoid pain.

This simple view always neglected many factors ever-present in human lives: the fear of losing honour, dignity and status, the distrust of change, the appeal of stability and familiarity. There was no place in it for more complex drives: vanity, fear of appearing vulnerable, the need to save face. Obsessed with material progress, the hyperrationalists ignored the lure of resentment for the left-behind, and the tenacious pleasures of victimhood.

But what makes resentment particularly malign today is a growing contradiction. The ideals of modern democracy – the equality of social conditions and individual empowerment – have never been more popular. But they have become more and more difficult, if not impossible, to actually realise in the grotesquely unequal societies created by our brand of globalised capitalism.

Issues of social justice and equality have receded along with conceptions of society or community – to be replaced by the freely choosing individual in the marketplace. According to the prevailing view today, the injustices entrenched by history or social circumstances cease to matter: the slumdog, too, can be a millionaire, and the individual's failure to escape the underclass is self-evident proof of his poor choices.

Never have so many free individuals felt so helpless – so desperate to take back control from anyone they can blame for their feeling of having lost it. It should not be surprising that we have seen an exponential rise in hatred of minorities, the main pathology induced by political and economic shocks." (adapted summary by me).

One of those economic shocks is the widening financial inequity worldwide. On 16 January 2017 Oxfam International published that on this planet eight men own the same wealth as the 3.6 billion people who make up the poorest half of humanity.[241]

Worldwide, nowadays we meet uprooted individuals who, alone, or inspired by a network of hate, did not participate enough in the societal progress. They are frustrated, or open to terrorist propaganda, destructive religious messages and false populist leaders. The thinking about "them" and "us" is influencing broad groups, leading to a fragmented and unhealthy society.

Our response from family medicine and primary care will have to be based on solidarity, on respect for diversity, on building bridges instead of walls, on establishing "connectedness". That is why the artwork on the cover of this book by Guy Timmerman is entitled "Interrelated Connectedness". That means that we have to choose for comprehensive solutions and new ways of living together, for empathy and for creating opportunities.

What Has Family Medicine and Primary Care to Offer in This Respect?

We have to offer a lot, provided we make the right choices at different levels.

At the **nano level** (individual interaction patient/citizen and provider): an open mind to listen to the needs, goals, anxieties, fears of the people we meet in primary care. Offering quality communication, creating the language and interaction people understand through a culture-sensitive approach. The importance of the encounter at the nano level cannot be overestimated: "*The core space of every health system is occupied by the unique encounter between one set of people who need services and another who have been entrusted to deliver them. This trust is earned through a special blend of technical competence and service orientation, steered by ethical commitment and social accountability, which forms the essence of professional work*".[97] The specificity of the primary care encounter is the generalist approach by professionals. In the context of the person with care needs, he is able to contribute in a tailored way to empowerment, treatment or solutions in the areas of life where this is necessary and desirable.[184] This will lead to comprehensive care and support securing a high quality of life for all citizens that enables them to take care of themselves at any time in life, to connect with social environment, and to maintain control over their lives with a view to optimise well-being and health. The starting point is a holistic concept of the human being. Mental, physical, social and ecological aspects of the person must always be approached in a coherent way. This reflects the eco-bio-psycho-social model. Family physicians and other primary care providers (nurses, social workers,...) will need the required knowledge, skills and attitudes to deal with complaints, worries and symptoms that very often are unspecified and require further exploration. Decision-making processes at this level will be characterised by uncertainty, working with hypotheses rather than fixed diagnoses, and shared decision processes. What we need are the "C"-words: Commitment, Connectedness, Clinical Competence, Cultural Competence,

Context, Comprehensiveness, Complexity, Co-ordination, Continuity and striking an appropriate balance between "Compassion" and "Computer".

At the **micro level** an integrated interprofessional approach by a co-operating team is essential to address the complexity of multi-problem situations, with the patients in the driver's seat, in order to contribute to the achievement of their goals. These interprofessional teams are organised as multidisciplinary practices (e.g. Community Health Centres), or as networks of different disciplines, using a shared Electronic Person Record. The team addresses the upstream causes of ill health, looking at housing, education, work,... linking with informal care givers and, when needed, facilitating development of social capital.[242] The approach by the team will be focusing on capabilities, not on deficiencies. The patient, together with the team, can take an advocacy role, signalising deficiencies in the care process or unhealthy social and environmental determinants.

At the **meso level** (the community) the primary care sector is accountable for health of a defined population. A typical size for a "Primary Care Zone" could be 100,000 population, but may vary according to local conditions. At this level the "health and social objectives" of the community should be reached, and well-functioning "Primary Care Zones" can be rewarded through e.g. an innovation grant. Access to care and addressing social determinants, organising continuity of care, organising continuous professional development of providers, taking care of professional and informal care givers, monitoring health indicators and quality of life,... can be important strategies at this level. Intersectoral action may contribute to strengthen social cohesion and to increase "interrelated connectedness".

This integrated community-based approach, in primary care, is completely different from the vertical disease-oriented programs that actually are prevailing in a lot of countries (programs for diabetes, HIV, hypertension,...) leading to fragmentation of care and entail the risk of "inequity by disease".[72] The primary care approach is integrating, is able to deal with multifaceted problems, and embraces complexity.

At this level integration between the local social policy and local health policy can reinforce the strength of primary care and its ability to tackle social inequities in health. This primary care approach also differs from the "syndemics"-approach, which has recently been presented as "completely innovative". The "syndemics"-approach provides a conceptual framework for understanding diseases or health conditions that arise in populations and that are exacerbated by the social, economic, environmental and political milieu in which a population is immersed. Of course, this is exactly what Community-Oriented Primary Care (see Chapter 2) is doing. But instead of looking at populations who live in the same community ("Primary Care Zone") the "syndemics"-approach looks at selections of the population who respond to a certain clustering of conditions, e.g. VIDDA (Violence, Immigration, Depression, Type 2 Diabetes and Abuse). "Syndemics" presents a "vertical" reductionist approach that once more will exclude people from service because they don't fit with the clustering acronyms.

There is a high risk that this "syndemics"-approach will have the same effect as the "selective primary health care" that was introduced in 1979, a year after the Alma-Ata Declaration (see Chapter 1), and that diverted resources and staff from generalist comprehensive primary care towards vertical disease-oriented (or in this case "clusters of problems"-oriented) programs.

Fortunately, the majority of academics in Public Health and Family Medicine/ Primary Care are convinced that the two disciplines have to co-operate to build strong and equitable health systems as was demonstrated at a joint side event at the World Health Assembly 2016 in Geneva with participation of WONCA, the World Federation of Public Health Associations (WFPHA), the European Forum for Primary Care (EFPC) and The Network: Towards Unity for Health. The Global Charter for the Public's Health[243] underpins this co-operation conceptually and Community-Oriented Primary Care[50] translates this into practice.

At the **macro level** strong primary health care systems are associated with a more equitable distribution of health in the population, as the late Barbara Starfield (Johns Hopkins, Baltimore, USA) documented,[244] and Kringos (University of Amsterdam, the Netherlands) provided evidence that in Europe strong primary care systems are associated with relatively lower socio-economic inequality, as measured by an indicator linking education levels to self-rated health.[245] Apart from its contribution to equity, there is increasing evidence that around one quarter of economic growth between 2000 and 2011 in low- and middle-income countries results from the value of improvements to health. The returns on investment in health are estimated to be 9 to 1. One extra year of life expectancy has been shown to raise Gross Domestic Product (GDP) per capita by about 4%. In countries with high fertility rates reduced likelihood of child mortality can positively influence household decisions on family planning. This contributes to a faster demographic transition and its associated economic benefits, often called the demographic dividend. According to the High-Level Commission on Health Employment and Economic Growth's report "Working for Health and Growth: Investing in the Health Workforce" investments in the health system also have multiplier effects that enhance inclusive economic growth, including via the creation of decent jobs. Targeted investment in health systems, including in the health workforce, promotes economic growth along other pathways: economic output, social protection and cohesion, innovation and health security.

The contribution of primary care to these developments is undeniable. Returns on investment in primary care are possible through job creation, strengthening gender and women's rights, investing in education, training and skills, keeping youngsters healthy in the community so that they can access education, health service delivery and organisation. Here the advice of the Commission is very clear: "Health Systems organised around clinical specialties will need to shift towards prevention and primary care".[246] Moreover, in order to reach Sustainable Development Goal n° 3, "Ensure healthy lives and promote well-being for all at all ages", primary care will strengthen the intersectoral action for health, involving domains described in the other 16 SDGs (promote justice, end poverty, encourage sustainable employment, promote peaceful communities).[247]

Other important economic returns on investment will come from increased cost-effectiveness when primary care is embedded in a gatekeeping system, where over 90% of the problems can be dealt with at the primary care level, and an appropriate selection of referrals increases the efficiency of the health system. Finally, the contribution of primary care to improve health of the people will increase their economic added value, and the positive impact of strong primary care on social cohesion will contribute to more "interrelated connectedness" in society.

In other words, there can be no excuse for politicians and other stakeholders for not increasing investments in family medicine and primary care.

How Can "Family Medicine" and Primary Care Make a Difference?

Adapting the work by John Gillies et al., the key-advantages of family medicine and primary care teams are:[248]

- *Trust*: the basis is high-quality empathic communication in the framework of good-quality care (see Chapter 6). Trust is essential for concordance with treatment, co-creation of health, effective gatekeeping, and avoidance of medicalisation (see Chapters 1 and 5), underpinned by local perceptions of altruism, fair dealing and other personal qualities, competence and integrity, and by both a rhetoric and an assumption of good intentions. Since 2016 an important component of trust, i.e. the perception that what somebody tells is the truth, has come into the societal debate. In a reflection on "Post-truth and science" Sir Michael Marmot (UCL, London, UK) notes: "*If we want the perceived dishonesty of the Trumps of the world and the Brexiteers to pass, then scientists and health professionals, for whom truth is central, have to be even more diligent. Remember whom the general public trust to tell the truth: nurses, doctors, teachers, judges, and scientists. The population and civilised values are on our side and the light will drive out the darkness*".[249]
- *Co-ordination*: bringing patients' multiple problems and issues into an integrated picture, co-ordination between patients and relatives, partners, between family physicians and other members of the primary health care team, social work, co-ordination between professionals and informal care givers, voluntary agencies, between hospital specialist and primary care services;
- *Continuity*: based on repeated contacts, strengthening a relationship with patients and citizens over months and years. Challenges integrate the fact that young providers, correctly, want a better balance between professional and private life.
- *Flexibility*: addressing problems according to degree of urgency and in the order and at the pace that suits patients; integrating professional, contextual and policy evidence; balancing individual and population approaches in day-to-day work, including Community-Oriented Primary

Care; liaising effectively with civil society organisations, actors from other sectors and local authorities, and being innovative.

- *Responsiveness*: family physicians in the context of primary care contact 90% of the population on the list over a 5-year period, including those who are "hard to reach". By doing so primary care can even reach homeless people[250] and other vulnerable groups for care and screening.
- *Advocacy*: by signalising problems in care provision, problems in access, and providing evidence about "upstream causes" (social, economic, environmental, housing, labour,...) to local, regional and national authorities.
- *Leadership*: focusing on implementation of change quickly, based on interprofessional knowledge and experience of local circumstances, supply and population characteristics. The longitudinal relationship of a primary care team with a population may contribute to strengthening the leadership role.

We Can Imagine It,
We Can Make It Happen

During the past 40 years, with different actors and involvement of the local population, we have been able to contribute to accessible integrated care in the community of Ledeberg in Ghent, to strengthen the focus on prevention and health promotion, to intersectoral action for health. Thanks to the collective efforts, in less than 20 years the community has been able to create "interrelated connectedness" whilst the number of nationalities in the neighbourhood increased from 20 to 106 nowadays. The presence of a multitude of care providers in the public, private not-for-profit sector and in private practices, all committed to their task, contributed to the fact that people nowadays, when they face a problem, know where to go, and that they are sure there is somebody available with an empathetic, listening ear. This largely strengthens social cohesion and stimulates connectedness. But perhaps the most important thing that happened was that this small community of 8,500 people that was "absorbed" by the city of Ghent in 1977, managed to get the attention of the Ghent policy-makers for its problems and challenges. In the future family medicine and primary care will have to take responsibility and contribute to advocacy in order to keep that attention.

As far as academic work is concerned, at Ghent University and also in the other Flemish universities, family medicine is now an established discipline, embedded in a primary care approach. Important research topics for the future are integrated care, task-shifting and competency sharing, use of ICT, and building primary care networks. Moreover, there is a need to strengthen the Primary Care Zones and to make sure that they are accountable for all the citizens on their territories: "Everybody counts!"

The concept of Goal-Oriented Care will be further explored and the same applies to the implementation of Community-Oriented Primary Care. Accessibility of Health Care and addressing social determinants of health will continue to be on the agenda.

The Way Forward

Apart from the destructive policy-developments in USA, there are positive signs: WHO is putting its commitment to primary care into practice, in different continents governments make a clear choice to build the health care systems on strong primary care, and the European Commission starts establishing a "European Pillar of Social Rights".[251]

Important values that underpin strong health care systems like social justice, solidarity,... are actually under pressure and fragmentation increases. There is a lack of trust and the antonym of trust is "fear", that shadows our societies today. Fear of terror. Fear of losing one's job. Fear of being poor. Fear of disease, fear of the Other. This pervasive feeling of fear suggests a sharp loss of trust in our culture, our institutions, even ourselves. As Richard Horton (*The Lancet*) recently wrote: "Loss of trust – the fear that wraps itself around us as a sincere response to danger – partly explains Europe's fracture, America's retreat, and the riots and rebellions afflicting some of the most disfigured nation-states. The expression of fear, together with its exploitation and manipulation by an unworthy political and media class, has given permission for (and possibly encouraged) unrestraint violence".[252] The answer can only be a strengthening of the political forces that challenge the fear and translate it into hope. Bernie Sanders states: "Making sure that every citizen has the right to child care, health care, a college education, and a secure retirement is not a radical idea. It is as American as apple pie. It will allow us to realise the ideals of the USA: that all of us are created equal – that we all have the right to life, liberty, and the pursuit of happiness".[253]

We need this hope to make sure that our grandchildren will have a sustainable future where they can develop their capabilities in a society based on solidarity, social justice, social cohesion and respect for diversity. I wish it for our five grandchildren – Jef, Wout, Lou, Flo, Niels – and for all the children in this world.

We can Imagine it, we can Make It Happen:

"Imagine there's no countries
It isn't hard to do,
Nothing to kill or die for
Not for religion, too
Imagine all the people
Living life in peace...

Imagine no possessions
I wonder if you can
No need for greed or hunger
A brotherhood of men
Imagine all the people
Sharing all the world...

You may say I'm a dreamer
But I'm not the only one
I hope some day you'll join us
And the world will live as one."

(adapted from John Lennon)

Reflection by Michael Marmot
Primary Care in Social Context

The West Midlands Fire Service invited me to spend a day with them in Birmingham, England. They had produced a report: "Improving Lives to Save Lives – Applying Marmot Principles". It was inspiring.

The core business of the Fire Service is putting out fires. Analogous to a good primary care centre, the fire service began to reach out to the community to prevent fires: smoke alarms, avoiding fire hazards in the home, and the like. They then began to go further. Make every contact count. They took my review of health inequalities in England, *Fair Society Healthy Lives: the Marmot Review*[254] as a basis for action to improve people's lives. The fire service worked with children, with older people, gave advice on housing. If a firefighter went into a house and suspected domestic violence, he or she did not say: that's someone else's job. They said: I am not equipped to deal with domestic violence, but I know who to contact, I know who is expert.

I went back to general practitioners in England and said: this is what firefighters are doing to address social determinants of health; what are you doing? I might have introduced them to Jan De Maeseneer. The kind of primary care that he has developed in Ghent, as laid out in this volume, has great potential to bridge the gap between primary care and social determinants of health.

There has been something of a chasm between primary care and public health. The one oriented to treating individuals, the other to improving population health. With my colleagues in the Institute of Health Equity, at UCL, we developed a five-fold plan for how doctors could address social determinants of health (http://www.instituteofhealthequity.org/Content/FileManager/wma-ihe-report_-doctors-for-health-equity-2016.pdf):

- Education and training
- See the patient in broader perspective
- Health service as employer – address conditions of work that affect health
- Working in partnership
- Advocacy

The future, as laid out in this book, is to bring these streams of work together. Further, we need to recognise that the way society is organised has profound impact, on psychosocial pathways, on health, and on health inequalities. Humane physicians such as Jan De Maeseneer, working in cross-disciplinary partnership, are key agents in improving societies for the benefits of all.

Michael Marmot is Director of the Institute of Health Equity at UCL. He chaired the WHO Commission on Social Determinants of Health, The Marmot Review of Health Inequalities in England, and the European Review of Social Determinants and the Health Divide. He is immediate Past President of the World Medical Association.

Epilogue

The Impossible Made Possible

How much can a man do? How many accomplishments are enough to consider a career "successful"? No doubt, the past four decades that have led to the material for this book are a series of extraordinary achievements. From health care provider to public polemicist, from academic researcher and teacher to advisor in innumerous boards: Professor De Maeseneer has excelled in the many commitments that he made, both on an individual basis with his work at the Community Health Centre Botermarkt at the core, as on a broader scale involving education and policy.

Not coincidentally, all chapters in this book begin with a testimony, taken from the everyday experiences that marked the past forty years. This rhetorical method is more than a literary gesture: it demonstrates the essence of the work Professor De Maeseneer has done throughout the years. A deeply rooted sense of human involvement has been at the core of his vigour to make change happen, from his early life as a student until the end of his academic tenure.

Looking back at the course of his life, one could believe that "interrelated connectedness" has been the motto of Professor De Maeseneer from the very beginning. In an era where primary care providers locked themselves up in their cabinet, he went into the outside world. Instead of adopting monodisciplinary medicine, he chose to develop a model for integrated primary care. Instead of accepting the impossible, he stood up, spoke up, and made the impossible possible. By means of collaboration, trust and persistence, he has put a definitive mark on primary care as it is today. Moreover, with "Together We Change" he has outlined the health care landscape of the future. Once again, the word "together" can't be coincidence.

Tomorrow Starts Today

Naturally, the work is never done. Shaping the future is an ongoing process, implementing dynamics that pop up in society, research, technology, science and so on. Throughout the chapters, several questions have risen both implicitly and explicitly. How will equity and accessibility for all be ensured? What does it mean to really put the patient at the centre of care? Can primary care appeal to investors? Are universities to be reformed to keep up with the complexity of the problems we face? Is there a way to bring research and real life closer together? Will students be able to cope with the growing amount of knowledge? To what extent should citizens be involved in decisions on the highest levels of care? When will the debate on the pros and cons of diverse payment systems be translated in policy decisions and actions? And what does it take to persuade international donors of the importance of strengthening horizontal primary health care systems in deprived regions all around the globe?

Surely, for every idea that has come to fruition, a question has arisen. Was it not Aristotle, one of the founding fathers of medicine, who remarked that "the more you know, the more you know you don't know"?

Looking at the next decades, the biggest challenge seems to be the ideological conflict between the neoliberal ideal of ultimate self-fulfillment opposed to the sense that connection between people is key to give meaning to one's life. In his artwork "Interrelated connectedness", Guy Timmerman has given birth to a symbiosis between individuality and collectivity, as if it were an artistic recipe for happiness. Within primary care organisation as it is today, maybe Community Health Centres can serve as a metaphor for the natural intersection between the self and the other?

Community Health Centres do not only originate from existing communities, they also maintain them. A feeling of interconnectedness must be supported by the notion that an interaction within a health care setting is provided free of charge and absolutely self-evident, or in other words: as an age-old instinct departing from humane commitment in relation to each other. In a century where even the most intuitive mutuality, i.e. the reciprocity between caregiver and patient, has been subjected to the laws of the free market, the Community Health Centres provide a model for a primary care that isn't hollowed out by the hegemony of cash and competition. On the contrary, these institutions can foster the idea of care-based communities as a hideout for a world where individuals are subject to constant comparison and mandatory self-enhancement – which are to be considered ingredients for a sheer rat race to misfortune.

Family Medicine and Primary Care

The Origin Of Change

I know that I speak for hundreds of colleagues when I express my deepest gratitude to Professor De Maeseneer for his endless investments in our training, his ongoing efforts to involve students in the design of the curriculum and his perseverance in implementing a socio-economic and ethical point of view throughout the bachelor and master years. Although he will no longer be the Head of the Department of Family Medicine and Primary Health Care at Ghent University, he will remain a role model for countless researchers, teachers, policy makers, activists and health care providers.

His conviction to always do the right thing, his profound trust that youngsters will make this world a better place and his confidence that justice will prevail, have set a remarkable example for the generations to come. Professor De Maeseneer has shown us the way forward, and so will his legacy in the forthcoming years.

The late James Baldwin once wrote that "the impossible is the least that one can demand". We are facing outbursts of terror, an overt propagation of less solidarity and less tolerability by political leaders whose extreme opinions become more and more mainstream, a widespread neoliberal logic that enslaves billions of people, a completely irrational denial of the ecological consequences of massive consumerism and a growing financial gap between a deprived majority and the happy few. Nowadays, there seems little room for hope. Nevertheless, consternation can be a catalysing force for change.

"A world that will live as one" can only be reached if the way is paved by the joined strength of many individuals. Indeed, the infeasible for a sole man is the common purpose of a whole movement. Out of the unthinkable, dreams are born. And out of dreams, a better world. Bearing Samuel Beckett's famous last lines of "The Unnamable" in mind, the only option is to embrace tomorrow through today's efforts. Whatever the odds, we will continue to pursue our imagination.

"I can't go on. I'll go on."

Jan-Jakob Delanoye, MD
Medical Student at Ghent University (2009-2016).
Trainee/resident in Family Medicine.
Member Young European Forum for Primary Care (You&EFPC).

Curriculum Vitae:
Professor Jan De Maeseneer

Background

Jan De Maeseneer (°1952, Ghent, Belgium) graduated as a Medical Doctor in 1977 at Ghent University. Since 1978 he has been working part-time as a family physician in the Community Health Centre Botermarkt in Ledeberg, in those days a deprived area in the city of Ghent. From 1978 to 1981 he worked also as a part-time research assistant in health promotion at the Department of Public Health (prof. K. Vuylsteek). In 1981 he became a part-time assistant at the Department of Family Medicine (prof. R. De Smet). From 1991 until 2017, he was Head of the Department. From 2008 until 2017, he served as the Vice-Dean for Strategic Planning at the Faculty of Medicine and Health Sciences.

Academic Career

Jan De Maeseneer is involved in undergraduate and postgraduate teaching, training and research. He was as president of the Educational Committee (from 1997 until 2016) in charge of a fundamental reform of the undergraduate curriculum (from a discipline-based towards an integrated contextual medical curriculum). This new curriculum was evaluated very positively by an international Accreditation Board and was awarded a Special Quality Award for its community orientation and social accountability in 2005.

Jan De Maeseneer is a member of the Board of Directors of the Inter-university Flemish Consortium for Vocational Training in Family Medicine. He has been chairing the Working Party for Family Medicine of the Belgian High Council for Medical Specialist and Family Physicians since 1998.

In 2004 Professor De Maeseneer received the "WONCA-Award for Excellence in Health Care: the Five-Star Doctor" at the 17th World Conference of Family Doctors in Orlando (USA). In 2008 he was awarded a "Doctor Honoris Causa"-degree at the Universidad Mayor de San Simon in Cochabamba (Bolivia). In

2010 he received the Price De Schaepdrijver-Caenepeel for developmental work from the Royal Flemish Academy of Medicine. Since 2011 he has been an honorary fellow of the Royal College of General Practitioners (UK) and an honorary member of the South-African Academy of Family Physicians. In 2014 he received a Special Award for Excellence in Health Professional Education at the Prince Mahidol Award Conference in Thailand. Since 2012 he has been a member of the Global Forum on Innovation of Health Professionals' Education at the National Academies of Sciences, Engineering and Medicine (Washington, USA). In 2015 he was holder of the Francqui Chair on Primary Care at the University of Antwerp (Belgium).

Research

The research activities are focused on: epidemiology of family practice, functioning of family physicians, prescription behaviour, medical decision-making, medical education, community-oriented primary care, health systems research, interprofessional teamwork, equity in health care, telematics in health care, health and poverty, health care in developing countries.

He wrote over 300 scientific publications leading to more than 4,000 citations. About 150 of the publications have been published in international journals with peer-review system (Web of Science). He also has given more than 130 lectures at national conferences and more than 170 lectures at international conferences. He is a member of the editorial board of the "*European Journal of General Practice*" and of "*BMC Family Practice*". For many years he has been active in the WICC (WONCA International Classification Committee), contributing to the development of the International Classification of Primary Care. Since October 2010 he has been Director of the International Centre for Primary Health Care and Family Medicine – Ghent University, a WHO Collaborating Centre on PHC.

Social Accountability

In 1990-1991 Jan De Maeseneer was advisor on primary health care of the federal Minister of Health in Belgium. Since 2010 he has been the Chairman of the Strategic Advisory Board of the Flemish Minister for Welfare, Health and Family, and has been president of the Health Council of the City of Ghent. He has been a member of the Advisory Committee on Medical Training of the EU and of the Scientific Advisory Board of the "Organisation for Accreditation and Quality Assurance" in Switzerland. From 2005 until 2017 Jan De Maeseneer was the Chairman of the European Forum of Primary Care (www.euprimarycare.org). From 2006 to 2008 he participated in the Knowledge Network on "Health Systems" of the WHO Commission on Social Determinants of Health. He is a member of the Primary Health Care Advisory Group, advising the WHO-European Regional Director in Copenhagen. He has been the Chairman of the Expert Panel on Effective Ways of Investing in Health (EXPH), advising the European Commission since 2013.

International Co-operation

Professor De Maeseneer has been involved in the development of various programs of international co-operation and student exchange (with University of Cochabamba – Bolivia, University of Cape Town – South-Africa, University Yaoundé I – Cameroon, University of Makerere – Kampala, University of Science and Technology in Mbarara – Uganda, University of Cuenca – Ecuador). He is promotor of the Primafamed-Network (www.primafamed. ugent.be). From 2007 till 2015 Jan De Maeseneer was the Secretary General of The Network: Towards Unity for Health (www.thenetworktufh.org). Since 2008 he has been a member of the Board of Directors of Global Health through Education, Training and Service (www.ghets.org). He is a member of the Lancet Commission on Primary Care in China.

Jan De Maeseneer is married to Anita De Winter (psychiatrist). They enjoy the company of two sons: Pieter and his partner Eefje, Daan and his partner Lies, and five grandchildren: Jef, Wout, Lou, Flo and Niels.

A personal note:

Prof. De Maeseneer was my head of department during all of the 23 years that I have been working at Ghent University. This above factual summing up of the different steps in his impressive career does not nearly reflect his true meaning for our department and for primary care in our country and abroad. Under his leadership the number of people working at our department has increased fivefold, research areas have expanded hugely, family medicine became an essential topic in undergraduate education and the quality of post-graduate training improved substantially. He was the inspirator and often architect of many of the policy changes that stimulated primary care in our country. His enthusiastic and well underpinned pleas for a comprehensive primary care and his contribution to the development of family medicine training all over the world has been an inspiration for a countless number of people in all levels of health care. But above all he was an excellent and inspiring boss, a wonderful person to work with, a leader who brought out the best in each of us.

Professor An De Sutter

Thanks

To my parents for giving us the opportunity to study in secondary school and to go to university, an opportunity that they did not have themselves. Thanks to my family for their support and understanding.

Thanks to the staff of the Community Health Centre Botermarkt – Ledeberg for their commitment, professionalism, feedback in the 40 years I had the privilege to work in the team and for the leadership of the Director General Leen De Roo. Thanks to the patients for their trust and sharing their stories.

Thanks to all who contributed in the last 40 years to providing care for the population in Ledeberg, for their commitment in the 3-monthly meetings of our "Platform", making a Community Diagnosis and acting accordingly. Thanks to the staff of the "Child and Family" Well Baby Clinic and the volunteers for their commitment.

Thanks to the Mayors and the Aldermen responsible in the City of Ghent for Health and Social Welfare, for taking the advice of the City Health Council seriously.

Thanks to the inspiring team that I had the opportunity to work with in the Department of Family Medicine and Primary Health Care at Ghent University: a special word of thanks to Claudine Lodomez, who has worked as my personal assistant for 23 years, processing a countless number of documents in Dutch, French, and English, including this book.

Thanks to the members of the Educational Committee and all those involved in the change process of the curriculum, especially the curriculum managers, for their vision, their enthusiasm. Special thanks to the thousands of students and the Student Working Group on Education whom I had the privilege to work with on their pathway towards becoming a care professional.

I also thank Ghent University and the Faculty of Medicine and Health Sciences for accepting me as a critical member of the academic community.

Thanks to the colleagues of the Departments of Family Medicine in Louvain, Antwerp and Brussels, for the 33 years we have already been building the project of a high quality vocational training for family medicine together. Special thanks to the general director Guy Gielis and to the general manager An Stockmans.

The different policy bodies that I was supporting as a member of advisory boards: at the Flemish level as the chair of the Strategic Advisory Board on Welfare, Health and Family; the Federal Planning Committee for Health Care Workforce; the High Council for Family Physicians and Specialists, advising the federal Minister of Health; and the Commission on Capitation Agreements for Community Health Centres/Medical Homes in the National Institute for Health and Disability Insurance (NIHDI), with special thanks to Dr De Ridder, Director-General Health Care.

I thank all the international organisations that I had the privilege to serve: The Network: Towards Unity for Health (Secretary General: 2007-2015); the European Forum for Primary Care (chairman: 2005-2017); the Expert Panel on Effective Ways of Investing in Health, advising the European Commission (chairman: 2013-today); the Primafamed Network (1997-today); WONCA (World Organisation of Family Doctors as an informal advisor); WHO Geneva and Copenhagen (Director International Centre for Primary Health Care and Family Medicine – Ghent University, WHO Collaborating Centre on PHC: 2010-today); the Lancet Commission on Primary Care in China (2016-today).

A special thanks to Pieter and Eefje, Daan and Lies, and their children Wout, Niels, Jef, Lou, Flo for their inspiration, their joy and for keeping me sharp.

Last but not least, I would like to thank my wife Anita: we started the journey together as family physicians, but as Kahlil Gibran said: "The oak tree and the cypress grow not in each other's shadow".[255] So, you decided to become a psychiatrist and to build a special career in that discipline. Thanks for your support and your continuous critical reflection. Without you all that is described in this book, could never have happened. **Thank you.**

List of Acronyms

ANC	African National Congress
BMS	Breast Milk Substitutes
CAS	Complex Adaptive Systems
CCM	Chronic Care Model
CHC	Community Health Centre
CME	Continuous Medical Education
COPC	Community Oriented Primary Care
COPD	Chronic Obstructive Pulmonary Disease
CSO	Civil Society Organisation
CT	Computerised Tomography
ECG	Electrocardiography
ECTS	European Credit Transfer System
EFPC	European Forum for Primary Care
EMA	European Medicines Agency
ENT	Ear-Nose-Throat
EXPH	Expert Panel on Effective Ways of Investing in Health (advising the European Commission)
FDA	Food and Drug Administration (USA)
FIC	Family of International Classifications
FP	Family Physician (in this book family physician and general practitioner are used interchangeably)
GDP	Gross Domestic Product
GHETS	Global Health through Education, Training and Service
GOBI-FFF	Growth monitoring, Oral rehydration techniques, Breastfeeding, Immunisation, Food supplementation, Female literacy, Family Planning
GP	General Practitioner (in this book general practitioner and family physician are used interchangeably)
HIV	Human Immunodeficiency Virus
ICD	International Classification of Diseases
ICF	International Classification of Function
ICFDH	International Classification of Functioning, Disability and Health
ICPC	International Classification of Primary Care

ICT	Information and Communication Technology
IPE	Interprofessional Education
ISDB	International Society of Drug Bulletins
LMICs	Low-Income and Middle-Income Countries
MPLA	Movement of the People for the Liberation of Angola
MRI	Magnetic Resonance Imaging
NCD	Non-Communicable Diseases
NGO	Non-Governmental Organisation
OECD	Organisation for Economic Co-operation and Development
PC	Primary Care
PCZ	Primary Care Zone
PHC	Primary Health Care
QOF	Quality and Outcomes Framework
QoL	Quality of Life
RCGP	Royal College of General Practitioners (UK)
RCPCH	Royal College of Paediatrics and Child Health (UK)
RCT	Randomised Controlled Trial
SAVA	Substance Abuse, Violence, and AIDS
SES	Socio-Economical Status
SWAPO	South West Africa People's Organisation
THEnet	Training for Health Equity Network
TINSTAAFL	There is no such thing as a free lunch
TUFH	Towards Unity For Health
VIDDA	Violence, Immigration, Depression, Type 2 Diabetes, and Abuse
VUCA	Volatile Uncertain Complex Ambiguous
WFPHA	World Federation of Public Health Associations
WHA	World Health Assembly
WHO	World Health Organisation
WHR	World Health Report
WONCA	World Organisation of Family Doctors

Endnotes

1 World Health Organisation/UNICEF. Primary Health Care: Report of the International Conference on Primary Health Care. Alma-Ata, USSR 6-12 September 1978. *Health for All Series*, n°1. Geneva: WHO, 1978. http://www.who.int/publications/almaata_declaration_en.pdf

2 Starfield, B. Is primary care essential? *The Lancet* 1994;344(8930):1129-33.

3 World Health Organisation. *The World Health Report 2008 — Primary Health Care, Now More Than Ever.* 2008. http://www.who.int/whr/2008/en

4 Kidd, M. (Ed.) *The Contribution of Family Medicine to Improving Health Systems: a Guidebook from the World Organization of Family Doctors.* 2nd edn. London, New York: Radcliffe Publishing, 2013.

5 CSDH. *Closing the Gap in a Generation: Health Equity through Action on the Social Determinants of Health. Final Report of the Commission on Social Determinants of Health. Geneva, World Health Organisation* (2008). Available at: http://www.who.int/social_determinants/final_report/csdh_finalreport_2008.pdf

6 De Maeseneer, J., van Weel C., Egilman, D., Mfenyana, K., Kaufman, A., Sewankambo, N., Flinkenflögel, M. Funding for primary health care in developing countries: money from disease specific projects could be used to strengthen primary care. *British Medical Journal* 2008;336:518-9.

7 De Lepeleire, J. Half a century of general practice: an interview-based exploration. *Tijdschr. voor Geneeskunde* 2012;68(20):1004-12.

8 Collings, J.S. General Practice in England today: Reconnaissance. *Lancet* 1950;(i)555-79.

9   Bitton, A., Ratcliffe, H.L., Veillard, J.H. et al. Primary Health Care as a Foundation for Strengthening Health Systems in Low- and Middle-Income Countries. *J Gen Intern Med* 2016.

10   Van der Werf, G., Zaat, J. The birth of an ideology: Woudschoten and family medicine. *Huisarts en Wetenschap* 2001;51(10):428-35 (in Dutch).

11   Querido, A. *Introduction to Comprehensive Health Care*. Lochem: De Tijdstroom, 1973 (in Dutch: reprint from 1955).

12   Illich, I. *Medical Nemesis: The Expropriation of Health*. London, Calder&Boyars, 1975.

13   Byrne, P., Long, B. *Doctors Talking to Patients*. HMSO: London, 1976.

14   Engel, G. The need for a new medical model: a challenge for biomedicine. *Science* 1977;196(4286): 129-36.

15   François, L., De Maeseneer, J. (Eds.). *Family Medicine at the Threshold of the 21st Century : Looking Back at the Future*. Ghent, Department of Family Medicine and PHC, 2000.

16   Sharmanov, T. *Almaty within the Context of the New Millennium of Human Evolution*. Ministry of Health of the Republic of Kazakhstan, Almaty, 2013.

17   Walsh, J.A., Warren, K.S. Selective Primary Health Care, an Interim Strategy for Disease Control in Developing Countries. *New England Journal of Medicine* 1979;301:967-74.

18   Cueto, M. The origins of primary health care and selective primary health care. *American Journal of Public Health* 2004;94(11):1864-74.

19   Newell, K.W. Selective Primary Health Care: the counter revolution. *Social Science and Medicine* 1988;26:903-6.

20   Nutting, P.A. *Community-Oriented Primary Care: from Principle to Practice*. Washington U.S. Department of Health and Human Services, 1987.

21   World Health Organisation. *The Ottawa Charter for Health Promotion.* Ottawa, 21 November 1986. Available at: http://www.who.int/ healthpromotion/conferences/previous/ottawa/en/

22   WICC. *International Classification of Primary Care.* Wonca (World Organisation of Family Doctors). Available at: http://wonca.net/site/ DefaultSite/filesystem/documents/Groups/WICC/International%20 Classification%20of%20Primary%20Care%20Dec16.pdf

23   De Maeseneer, J. *Family Medicine: an Exploration. An Exploratory Research with GP-Preceptors at Ghent University.* Ghent University, 1989 (in Dutch). Available at: https://biblio.ugent.be/publication/8514435/file/8514436. pdf

24   Mold, J.W., Blake, G.H., Becker, L.A. Goal-Oriented Medical Care. *Family Medicine* 1991;23:46-51.

25   Guyatt, G., Cairns, J., Churchill, D. et al. Evidence-Based Medicine: a new approach to teaching the practice of medicine. *JAMA* 1992;268(17):2420-25.

26   Sackett, D.L., Rosenberg, W.M.C., Muir Gray, J.A., Haynes, R.B., Richardson, W.S. Evidence Based Medicine: what it is and what it isn't. *BMJ* 1996;312:71.

27   De Maeseneer, J.M., van Driel, M.L., Green, L.A., van Weel, C. The Need for Research in Primary Care. *Lancet* 2003;362:1314-9.

28   Flinkenflögel, M., Essuman, A., Chege, P., Ayankogbe, O., De Maeseneer, J. Family Medicine training in sub-Saharan Africa: South-South co-operation in the Primafamed project as strategy for development. *Fam Pract* 2014;31(4):427-38.

29   Marmot, M., Shipley, M., Rose, G. Inequalities in death – specific explanations of a general pattern? *Lancet* 1984;i:1003-6.

30   Marmot, M., Davey Smith, G., Stansfeld, S., et al. Health Inequalities among British Civil Servants: the Whitehall II Study. *Lancet* 1991;337:1387-93.

31   Mackenbach, J.P., van de Mheen, H., Stronks, K. A prospective cohort study investigating the explanation of socio-economic inequalities in health in the Netherlands. *Soc Sci Med* 1994;38(2):299-308.

32   *Commission on Social Determinants of Health.* Geneva, World Health Organisation, 2008. Available on: http://apps.who.int/iris/bitstream/10665/69832/1/WHO_IER_CSDH_08.1_eng.pdf

33   World Health Organisation. *Primary Health Care: Now More Than Ever!* Geneva, World Health Organisation 2008. Available at: http://www.who.int/whr/2008/whr08_en.pdf

34   Barnett, K., Mercer, S.W., Norbury, M. et al. Epidemiology of multi-morbidity and implications for health care, research and medical education: a cross-sectional study. *Lancet* 2012;380:37-43.

35   Kidd, M. *The Contribution of Family Medicine to Improving Health Systems. A Guidebook from the World Organisation of Family Doctors.* London, Radcliffe Publishing, 2013.

36   *High-Level Commission on Health Employment and Economic Growth: Working for Health and Growth: Investing in the Health Workforce.* Geneva, World Health Organization 2016. Available at: http://apps.who.int/iris/bitstream/10665/250047/1/9789241511308-eng.pdf?ua=1

37   OECD. *Caring for Quality in Health: Lessons Learned from 15 Reviews of Health Care Quality.* OECD Reviews of Health Care Quality, OECD Publishing Paris, 2017. Available at: http://dx.doi.org/10.1787/9789264267787-en

38   EXPH (Expert Panel on Effective Ways of Investing in Health). *Report on Definition of a Frame of Reference in Relation to Primary Care with a Special Emphasis on Financing Systems and Referral Systems.* Brussels, 10 July 2014. Available at: http://ec.europa.eu/health/expert_panel/sites/expertpanel/files/004_definitionprimarycare_en.pdf

39   Ginsburg, O., Bray, F., Coleman, M.P. et al. Health, Equity and Women's cancers 1: The global burden of women's cancers: a grant challenge in global health. *Lancet* 2017;389:847-60.

40   Engels, F. *Condition of the Working Class in England.* Leipzich, 1845 (in German); New York, London 1887 (English edition). Available at: https://www.marxists.org/archive/marx/works/download/pdf/condition-working-class-england.pdf

41   Morley, I. City Chaos, Contagion, Chadwick and Social Justice. Yale J *Biol Med* 2007;80(2):61-72.

42   Mackenbach, J.P. Politics is nothing but medicine at a larger scale: reflections on public health's biggest idea. *J Epidemiol Community Health* 2009;63(3):181-4.

43   Marmot, M.G., Stansfeld, S., Patel, C. et al. Health Inequalities among British Civil Servants: the Whitehall II Study. *Lancet* 1991;337(8754):1387-93.

44   Hart, J.T. The Inverse Care Law. *Lancet* 1971;297(7696):405-12.

45   Willems, S. *The Socio-Economic Gradient in Health: a Never-ending Story? A Descriptive and Explorative Study in Belgium.* Ghent, Department of Family Medicine and Primary Health Care, 2005.

46   Starfield, B. *Primary Care. Balancing Health Needs, Services and Technology.* Oxford, Oxford University Press, 1998, 404.

47   De Maeseneer, J., Willems, S., De Sutter, A., Van de Geuchte, M.L., Billings, M. *Primary Health Care as a Strategy for Achieving Equitable Care: a Literature Review Commissioned by the Health Systems Knowledge Network.* Ghent University, Department of Family Medicine and Primary Health Care, 2007. Available at: www.who.int/social_determinants/resources/csdh_media/primary_health_care_2007_en.pdf

48 Haggerty, J.L., Lévesque, J.F., Hogg, W., Wong, S. The strength of Primary Care Systems. Stronger systems improve population health but require higher levels of spending. *BMJ* 2013;346:3777.

49 Kringos, D.S., Boerma, W., van der Zee, J., Groenewegen, P. Europe's strong primary care systems are linked to better population health but also to higher health spending. *Health Affairs* 2012;32:686-94.

50 Rhyne, R., Bogue, R., Kukulka, G,. Fulmer, H. (Eds.) *Community-oriented Primary Care: Health Care for the 21st Century.* Washington, DC: American Public Health Association, 1998.

51 Pickles, W.N. *Epidemiology in Country-practice.* London: The Devonshire Press (Ltd.) reissued, 1972.

52 Tollman, S.M. The Pholela Health Centre – The Origins of Community-Oriented Primary Health Care (COPC). An appreciation of the work of Sidney and Emily Kark. *S Afr Med J* 1994;84(10):653-58.

53 Willems, S., Vanobbergen, J., Martens, L., De Maeseneer, J. The independent impact of household- and neighbourhood-based social determinants on early childhood caries. A cross-sectional study of inner-city children. *Fam Community Health* 2005;28(2):168-75.

54 Smits, F.T.M. Frequent attenders: how frequent, who and why? Huisarts Wet-2015;58(7):358-61 (in Dutch).

55 Hart L, Horton R. Syndemics: committing to a healthier future. *Lancet* 2007;389:888-89.

56 Rechel, B., Mladovsky, P., Ingleby, D., Mackenbach, J. P., & McKee, M. Migration and health in an increasingly diverse Europe. *Lancet* 2013;381(9873), 1235-45.

57 Napier, A.D., Ancarno, C., Butler, B., Calabrese, J., Chater, A., Chatterjee, H. Woolf, K. Culture and health. *Lancet* 2014;384(9954):1607-39.

58 Suess, A., Ruiz Perez, I., Ruiz Azarola, A., & March Cerda, J.C. The right of access to health care for undocumented migrants: a revision of comparative analysis in the European context. *Eur J Public Health* 2014;24(5):712-20.

59 Watt G. *General Practitioners at the Deep End. The experience and views of general practitioners working in the most severely deprived areas of Scotland.* London, Royal College of General Practitioners, Occasional Paper 89, 2012.

60 Bodenheimer, T., Sinsky, C. From triple to quadruple aim: care of the patient requires care of the provider. *Ann Fam Med* 2004;12:573-576.

61 The Marmot Review. *Fair Society, Healthy Lives.* London, the Marmot Review 2010.

62 Verlinde, E., Verdée, T., Van de Walle, M., Art, B., De Maeseneer, J., Willems, S. Unique Health Care Utilization Patterns in a Homeless Population in Ghent. *BMC Health Services Research* 2010;10:242.

63 Wilkinson, R., Pickett, K. *The Spirit Level. Why Greater Equality Makes Societies Stronger.* London, Bloomsburg Press, 2010.

64 Dickman, S.L., Himmelstein, D.U., Woolhandler, S. America: equity and equality in health 1. Inequality and the health-care system in the USA. *Lancet* 2017;389:1431-41.

65 Sanders, B. An agenda to fight inequality. *Lancet* 2017;389:1376-7.

66 Institute of Medicine; Committee on Population; Board on Population Health and Public Health Practice; Panel on Understanding Cross-National Health Differences Among High-Income Countries; Woolf, S.H., Laudan, A. (Eds.) *US Health in International Perspective: Shorter Lives, Poorer Health.* Washington, DC: National Academies Press, 2013.

67 Woolhandler, S., Himmelstein, D.U. Single-payer reform: the only way to fulfill the president's pledge of more coverage, better benefits, and lower costs. *Ann Intern Med* 2017: published online Feb 21.

68   Anonymous. What has Europe ever done for health? *Lancet* 2017;389:1165.

69   European Commission. *Communication from the Commission to the European Parliament, the Council, The European and Social Committee and the Committee of the Regions: Establishing a European Pillar of Social Rights.* Brussels, European Commission, 26.04.2017.

70   De Maeseneer, J., Boeckxstaens, P. James Mackenzie Lecture 2011: Multimorbidity, Goal-Oriented Care and Equity. *Br J Gen Pract* 2012;62:522-4.

71   Sixty-Second World Health Assembly. Resolution WHA62.12. *Primary health care, including health system strengthening.* May 22, 2009. Available at http://www.who.int/hrh/resources/A62_12_EN.pdf

72   De Maeseneer, J., Roberts, R.G., Demarzo, M., Heath, I., Sewankambo, N., Kidd, M.R., van Weel, C., Egilman, D., Boelen, C., Willems, S. Tackling NCDs: A different approach is needed. *Lancet* 2011; 379(9829):1860-1.

73   WHO. *Mortality and Burden of Disease Estimates for WHO Member States in 2008.* Geneva: World Health Organisation, 2010.

74   Anderson, G., Horvath, J. *Chronic Conditions: Making the Case for Ongoing Care.* Baltimore, MD: Johns Hopkins University, 2002.

75   Mannino, D.M., Thorn, D., Swensen, A., Holguin, F. Prevalence and outcomes of diabetes, hypertension and cardiovascular disease in COPD. *Eur Respir J* 2008;32:962-9.

76   Barnett, K., Mercer, S.W., Norbury, M., Watt, G., Byke, S., Guthrie, B. Epidemiology of multimorbidity and implications for health care, research and medical education: a cross-sectional study. *Lancet* 2012;380:37-43.

77   Braithwaite, R.S., Justice, A.C., Chang, C.C. et al. Estimating the proportion of patients infected with HIV who will die of comorbid diseases. *Am J Med* 2005; 118:890-98.

78   Friss-Moller, N., Sabin, C.A., Weber, R. et al. Combination antiretroviral therapy and the risk of myocardial infarction. *N Engl J Med* 2003;348:1993-2003.

79   Vance, D.E., Mugavero, M., Willig, J., Raper, J.L., Saag, M.S. Aging with HIV : a cross sectional study of comorbidity prevalence and clinical characteristics across decades of life. *J Assoc Nurses AIDS Care* 2011;22(1): 17-25.

80   Crothers, K., Butt, A.A., Gibert, C.L. et al. Increased COPD among HIV positive compared to HIV negative veterans. *Chest* 2006; 130: 1326-33.

81   Gillam, S., Siriwardena, N. *The Quality and Outcomes Framework. QOF-transforming general practice.* Oxford: Radcliffe, 2011.

82   Norbury, M., Fawkes, N., Guthrie, B. Impact of the GP contract on inequalities associated with influenza immunisation: a retrospective population-database analysis. *British Journal of General Practice* 2011;61(588): e379-e385.

83   Boeckxstaens, P., De Smedt, D., De Maeseneer, J., Annemans, L., Willems, S. The equity dimension in the Quality and Outcomes Framework. A systematic Review. *BMC Health Services Research* 2011;31(1):209.

84   Heath, I., Rubinstein, A., van Driel, M.L. et al. Quality in primary health care: a multidimensional approach to complexity. *BMJ* 2009;338:911-3.

85   Wagner, E.H. Chronic disease management. What will it take to improve care for chronic illness? *Eff Clin Pract* 1998;1:2-4 .

86   Boyd, C.M., Darer, J., Boult, C., Fried, L.P., Boult, L., Wu, A.W. Clinical practice guidelines and quality of care for older patients with multiple comorbid diseases. *JAMA* 2005;294:716-24.

87   WHO. *International Classification of Functioning and Disability in Health (ICF).* Geneva, WHO, 2001. Available at http:///www.who.int/classifications/icf/en/

88   Boeckxstaens, P., Lanssens, M., Decuypere, C., Brusselle, G., Kuehlein, T., De Maeseneer, J., De Sutter, A. A qualitative interpretation of challenges associated with helping patients with multiple chronic diseases identified their goals. *Journal of Comorbidity* 2016;6(2).

89   Mendenhall, E. Syndemics: a new path for global health research. *Lancet* 2017;389:889-91.

90   Starfield, B. The hidden inequity in health care. *Int Journal for Equity in Health* 2011;10:15.

91   Swanson, R.C., Mosley, H., Sanders, D. et al. Call for global health-systems impact assessments. *Lancet* 2009;374:433-5.

92   Johnson, D., Saavedra, P., Sun, E. et al. Community Health Workers and Medicaid Managed Care in New Mexico. *J Community Health* 2012;37(3):563-71.

93   De Maeseneer, J., Willems, S., De Sutter, A., Van De Geuchte, M.L., Billings. *Primary health care as a strategy to achieve equitable care: a literature review commissioned by the Health Systems Knowledge Network*. Geneva: World Health Organization, 2007. http://www.who.int/social_determinants/resources/csdh_media/primary_health_care_2007_en.pdf

94   Pendleton, D.A. *Doctor Patient Communication*. Doctoral dissertation, University of Oxford, 1981.

95   SARWGG. *New Professionalism in care and support as a task for the future*. Brussels, Strategic Advisory Board Welfare, Health and Family, 2015. Available at: http://www.sarwgg.be/sites/default/files/documenten/SARWGG_20151217_New%20Professionalism_Vision%20statement_DEF.pdf

96   Anonymous. *Guiding Patients through Complexity: Modern Medical Generalism*. London, Report of an independent commission for the Royal College of General Practitioners and the Health Foundation; October 2011.

97 Frenk, J., Chen, L., Bhutta, Z.A., et al. Health professionals for a new century: transforming education to strengthen health systems in an interdependent world. *Lancet* 2010;376:1923-58.

98 Kohn, L.T., Corrigan, J.M., Donaldson, M.S. (Eds.) *To Err Is Human.* Washington, National Academy Press, 1999.

99 Sackett, D.L., Haynes, R.B., Tugwell, P. *Clinical Epidemiology: a Basic Science for Clinical Medicine.* Boston, Little Brown and Company, 1985.

100 Elstein, A.S., Schulman, L.S., Sprafka, S.A. *Medical Problems Solving: An Analysis of Clinical Reasoning.* Cambridge, MA: Harvard University Press, 1978.

101 Gruppen, L.D., Woolliscroft, J.O., Wolf, F.M. The contribution of different components of the clinical encounter in generating and eliminating diagnostic hypotheses. *Res Med Educ* 1988;27:242-7.

102 Stolper, E., van Bokhoven, M., Houben, P., Van Royen, P., van de Wiel, M., van der Weijden, T., Dinant, G.J. The diagnostic role of gut feelings in general practice: a focus group study of the concept and its determinants. *BMC Family Practice* 2009;10:17.

103 Buntinx, F. et al. *Pijn op de borst (chest pain).* Louvain, Academic Centre for Family Medicine, 1988.

104 Norman, G.R., Monteiro, S.D., Sherbino, J., Ilgen, J.S., Schmidt, H.G., Mamede, S. The causes of errors in clinical reasoning: cognitive biases, knowledge deficits and dual process thinking. *Acad Med* 2017;92:23-30.

105 Kahneman, D. *Thinking, Fast and Slow.* U.S., Farrar, Straus and Giroux, 2011.

106 Mc Grayne, S.B. *The Theory That Would Not Die. How Bayes' Rule Cracked the Enigma Code, Hunted Down Russian Submarines and Emerged Triumphant from 2 Centuries of Controversy.* New Haven, London, Yale University Press, 2011.

107 Stolper, E., van de Wiel, M., Van Royen, P., Van Bokhoven, M., van der Weijden, T., Dinant, G.J. Gut feelings as third track in general practicioners' diagnostic reasoning. *J Gen Intern Med* 2010;26(2):197-203.

108 Toulmin, S. On the nature of the physicians' understanding. *J Med Philos* 1976;1:32-50.

109 Montgomery, K. *How Doctors Think. Clinical Judgement and a Practice of Medicine*. Oxford, New York: Oxford University Press, 2006.

110 Raffle, A.E., et al. Outcomes of screening to prevent cancer: analysis of cumulative incidence of cervical abnormality and modelling of cases and deaths prevented. *BMJ* 2003;326(7395):901.

111 Taylor, F., et al. *Statins for the primary prevention of cardiovascular disease.* Cochrane Database of Systematic Reviews, 2013(1).

112 Saquib, N., Saquib, J., Ionnadis, J.P. Does screening for disease save lives in asymptomatic adults? Systematic review of meta-analyses and randomized trials. *International Journal of Epidemiology* 2015;44(1):264-77.

113 Welch, H.G., Black, W.C. Overdiagnosis in cancer. *J Natl Cancer Inst* 2010;102(9):605-13.

114 Getz, L., Sigurdsson, J.A., Hetlevik, I. Is opportunistic disease prevention in the consultation ethically justifiable? *BMJ* 2003;327(7413):498-500.

115 Starfield B, Hyde J, Gervas J, Heath I. The concept of prevention: a good idea gone astray? *J Epidemiol Community Health* 2008;62:580-3.

116 Jamoulle, M. Quaternary prevention, an answer of family doctors to overmedicalisation. *Int J Health Policy Manag* 2015;2:61-4.

117 Science Museum. *Brought to life: exploring the history of medicine: Thalidomide.* Available at: http://www.sciencemuseum.org.uk/broughttolife/themes/controversies/thalidomide

118   International Society of Drug Bulletins. *ISDB information booklet: Independence from drug companies is a key element of our policy.* Verona, Italy, International Society of Drug Bulletins, 2008. Available at: www.isdbweb.org/documents/uploads/Manual/ ISDBBooklet2008EnglishUpdate_000.pdf

119   Minerva. *Tijdschrift voor Evidence-Based Medicine. (Journal for Evidence-Based Medicine: in Dutch)* Ghent, University Hospital, 6K3. Available at: http://www.minerva-ebm.be/Home/Contact

120   De Meyere, M. *Acute keelpijn in de eerstelijn (Acute sore throat in primary care).* Ghent, Department of Family Medicine and Primary Health Care, 1990.

121   Christiaens, T., De Meyere ,M., Verschraegen, G., Peersman, W., Heytens, S., De Maeseneer, J. Randomised controlled trial of nitrofurantoin versus placebo in the treatment of uncomplicated urinary tract infection in adult women. *British Journal of General Practice* 2002;52:729-34.

122   De Sutter, A., De Meyere, M., Christiaens, T., van Driel, M., Peersman, W., De Maeseneer, J. Does Amoxicillin improve outcomes in patients with purulent rhinorrhea? A pragmatic randomised double-blind control trial in family practice. *J Fam Pract* 2002;51:317-23.

123   van Driel, M., Coenen, S., Dirven, K., Lobbestael, J., Janssens, I., Van Royen, P., Haaijer-Ruskamp, F.M., De Meyere, M., De Maeseneer, J., Christiaens, T. What is the role of quality circles in strategies to optimise antibiotic prescribing? A pragmatic cluster-randomised control trial in primary care. *Qual Saf Health Care* 2007;16(3):197-202.

124   van Driel, M., De Sutter, A., Deveugele, M., Peersman, W., Butler, C.C., De Meyere, M., De Maeseneer, J., Christiaens, T. Are sore throat patients who hope for antibiotics actually asking for pain relief? *Ann Fam Med* 2007;4:494-9.

125   Hickner, J. A new look at an old problem: inappropriate antibiotics for acute respiratory infections. *Ann Fam Med* 2006;4: 484-5.

126 Goldacre, B. *Bad pharma: how drug companies misled the doctors and harm patients*. London, Fourth Estate, 2012.

127 DeJong, C., Aguilar, T., Tseng, C.W. et al. Pharmaceutical industry-sponsored meals and physician prescribing patterns for Medicare beneficiaries. *JAMA Intern Med* 2016;176(8):1114-22.

128 Moynihan, R. The making of a disease: female sexual dysfunction. *BMJ* 2003;326:45.

129 Pharma.be. *Deontological code (in Dutch)*. Available at: http://www.pharma.be/nl/pharma-be/deontologische-code.html

130 Gulland, A. Royal College told to stop taking money from infant formula milk firms. *BMJ* 2016;353:i2459.

131 Modi, N., et al. Health Professional Associations and Industry Funding – Reply from Modi et al. *Lancet* 2017;389:1693-4.

132 O'Brien, D. Health Professional Associations and Industry Funding – Reply from O'brien. *Lancet* 2017;389:1694.

133 Forsyth, S. Health Professional Associations and Industry Funding-Reply from Forsyth. *Lancet* 2017;389:1694-5.

134 Waterston, T., et al. Health Professional Associations and Industry Funding – Reply from Waterston et al. *Lancet* 2017;389:1695.

135 Savage, F. Health Professional Associations and Industry Funding – Reply from Savage. *Lancet* 2017;389:16-96.

136 Supreme Court of Texas. *Abbott Laboratories, Inc. v. Segura*. 907 S.W.2d 503.1995. https://scholar.google.com/scholar_case?case=1889018415231 032770&hl=en&as_sdt=6&as_vis=1&oi=scholarr.

137 Parry, K.C. Health Professional Association and Industry Funding – Reply from Parry et al. *Lancet* 2017;389:1696.

138   Forbes. *Fortune 500 Industries*. 2016. http://money.cnn_com/magazines/
       fortune/fortune500/

139   Mazzucato, M. *Contribution to the UN High-Level Panel on Access to
       Medicines*. Sussex, UK, Science Policy Research Unit, University of
       Sussex, 28 February 2016. Available: http://www.unsgaccessmeds.org/
       inbox/2016/2/28/mariana-mazzucato

140   Mazzucato, M. *The Entrepreneurial State: Debunking Public versus Private
       Sector Myths*. London, UK, Anthem Press, 2013. US Edition (Public
       Affairs 2015).

141   Vallas, S.P., Kleinman, D., Biscotti, D., Block and Keller (Eds.), *Political
       Structures and the Making of US Biotechnology*, 2011.

142   Expert Panel on Effective Ways of Investing in Health (EXPH). *Report
       on Access to Health Services in the European Union*, Brussels, EXPH, 3
       May 2016. Available at: https://ec.europa.eu/health/expert_panel/sites/
       expertpanel/files/015_access_healthservices_en.pdf

143   Lepage-Nefkens, I., Douw, K., Mantjes, G., de Graaf, G., Leroy, R.,
       Cleemput, I. *Horizon Scanning for Pharmaceuticals: Proposal for the
       BeNeLuxA Collaboration. Health Services Research (HSR)*. Brussels:
       Belgian Health Care Knowledge Center (KCE). 2017. KCE Report 283.
       D/2017/10.273/15. Available at: https://kce.fgov.be/sites/default/files/
       page_documents/Horizon%20scanning_ScientificReport_.pdf

144   Huffman, M.D., Xavier, D., Perel, P. Uses of polypills for cardiovascular
       disease and evidence to date. *Lancet* 2017;389:1055-65.

145   Webster, R., Castellano, J.M., Onuma, O.K. Putting polypills into practice:
       challenges and lessons learned. *Lancet* 2017;389:1066-74.

146   Balarajan, Y., Selvaraj, S., Subramanian, S.V. Health care and equity in
       India. *Lancet* 2011:377;505-15.

147   Cochrane AL. *Effectiveness and Efficiency: Random Reflections on Health
       Services*. London: Nuffield Provincial Hospitals Trust, 1972.

148 Lohr, K.M. *Medicare: a Strategy for Quality Assurance*. Washington DC: National Academy Press, 1990.

149 Donabedian, A. The quality of care. How can it be assessed? *JAMA* 1988; 260:1743-8.

150 De Maeseneer, J. De zorg voor de kwaliteit en de kwaliteit van de zorg [The care for quality and the quality of care]. *Huisarts Wet* 1993; 36:437-39.

151 van Weel, C. Examination of context of medicine. *Lancet* 2001;357:733.

152 World Health Organisation, *International Classification of Functioning, Disability and Health*. Geneva, World Health Organisation, 2001. Available at: www.who.int/classifications/icf/en/

153 van Weel, C. Chronic diseases in general practice: the longitudinal dimension. *Eur J Gen Pract* 1996;2:17-21.

154 De Meyere, M., Mervielde, J., Verschraegen, G., Bogaert, M. Effect of penicillin on the clinical course of streptococcal pharyngitis in general practice. *Eur J Clin Pharmacol* 1992; 43: 581-5.

155 MacKay, D.M. Treatment of acute bronchitis in adults without underlying disease. J Gen Intern Med 1996; 11: 557-62.

156 Richards, J.P. Evidence based general practice. *BMJ* 1997; 314: 525.

157 Bodenheimer, T. Uneasy alliance: clinical investigators and the pharmaceutical industry. *N Engl J Med* 2000; 342: 1539-44.

158 Ong, L.M.L., de Haes, J.C.J.M., Hoos, A.M., Lammes, F.B. Doctor-patientcommunication: a review of literature. *Soc Sci Med* 1995; 40: 903-18.

159 Deveugele, M., Derese, A., van den Brink, A., Bensing, J., De Maeseneer, J. Consultation length in general practice: cross sectional study in six European countries. *BMJ* 2002; 325: 472-7.

160 Sunaert, P., Feyen, L., De Maeseneer, J. Inclusie, exclusie en uitval in relatie tot demografische en sociale economische kenmerken. [Inclusion, exclusion and drop-out in relation to demographic and socio-economic characteristics.] *Huisarts Wet* 1998; 41: 193-5.

161 Wallston, B.S., Wallston, K.A, Kaplan, G.D., Maides, S.A. Development and Validation of the Health Locus of Control (HLC) Scale. *J Consult Clin Psychology* 1976;44(4):580-5.

162 Ramsey, S.D. Suboptimal medical therapy in COPD: exploring the causes and consequences. *Chest* 2000;117:335-75.

163 Maynard, A. Evidence based medicine: an incomplete method for informing treatment choices. *Lancet* 1997;349:126-8.

164 Expert Panel on Effective Ways of Investing in Health (EXPH). *Final report on future EU agenda on quality of health care with a special emphasis on patient safety.* Brussels, EXPH, 9 October 2014. Available at: http://ec.europa.eu/health/expert_panel/sites/expertpanel/files/006_safety_quality_of_care_en.pdf

165 Grol, R. *Implementing Change in Primary Care. On the Trail of Better Quality. In: De Lepeleire J (ed). Back to the Future. Reflections on General Practice in a Changing World.* Antwerpen, Garant, 2008.

166 Braspenning, J.C.C., Pijnenborg, L., In 't Veld, C.J., Grol, R.P.T.M. (Eds). *Working for Quality in Family Practice. Indicators Based on the NHG-Guidelines.* Houten, Bohn Stafleu Van Loghum, 2005.

167 Goderis, G., Borgermans, L., Heyrman, J., Van Den Broeke, C., Grol, R., Boland, B., Mathieu, C. Type 2 diabetes in primary care in Belgium: need for structured shared care. *Exp Clin Endocrinol Diabetes* 2009;117:1-6.

168 Flottorp, S., Havelsrud, K., Oxman, A. Process evaluation of a cluster randomised trial of tailored interventions to implement guidelines in primary care – why is it so hard to change practice? *Fam Pract* 2003;20(3):333-9.

169 Equip (WONCA). Equity, a core dimension of quality of primary care: draft document. *Equip*, 05.02.2016.

170 Weber, M. *Die protestantische Ethik und der "Geist" des Kapitalismus*. New edition by Lichtblau K and Weiß J. Wiesbaden, Springer Fachmedien, 2016.

171 Deschepper, R., Vander Stichele, R.H., Haaijer-Ruskamp, F.M. Cross-cultural differences in lay attitudes and utilisation of antibiotics in a Belgian and a Dutch city. *Patient Education in Counseling* 2002;48(2):161-9.

172 Miller, G.E. The assessment of clinical skills/competence/performance. *Academic Medicine* 1990;65(9): S63-7.

173 Boelen, C. Medical Education Reform: the need for global action. *Academic Medicine* 1992;67:745-9.

174 Boelen, C. The Five-Star Doctor: an asset to health care reform? *Hum Resour Dev J*, 1997;1.available at: http://www.who.int/hrh/en/HRDJ_1_1_02.pdf

175 Deveugele, M., Derese, A., De Maesschalck, S., Willems, S., van Driel, M., De Maeseneer, J. Teaching communication skills to medical students, a challenge in the curriculum? *Patient Educ Couns* 2005;58:265-70.

176 Art, B., De Roo, L., Willems, S., De Maeseneer, J. An Interdisciplinary Community Diagnosis Experience in an Undergraduate Medical Curriculum: Development at Ghent University. *Academic Medicine* 2008;83(7): 675-83.

177 Cruess, R.L., Cruess, S.R., Steinert, Y. Amending Miller's Pyramid to include Professional Identity Formation. *Acad Med* 2016;91:180-5.

178 VLIR. De Onderwijsvisitatie Geneeskunde. *Evaluatie van de kwaliteit van de opleidingen geneeskunde aan de Vlaamse Universiteiten. [An assessment of the quality of undergraduate medical training programs in the Flemish universities]*. Brussels, December 2005 (in Dutch). Available at: http://

www.vlir.be/media/docs/Visitatierapporten/2005/kv05v2-geneeskunde.
pdf

179 Van der Veken, J,. Valcke, M., et al. The Potential of the Inventory of
Learning Styles to Study Students' Learning Patterns in Three Types of
Medical Curricula. *Medical Teacher* 2008;30:(9-10): 863-9.

180 Van der Veken, J., Valcke, M., De Maeseneer, J., Derese, A. Impact of
the transition from a conventional to an integrated contextual medical
curriculum on students' learning patterns: A longitudinal study. *Medical
Teacher* 2008; 31(5):433-41.

181 Van der Veken, J., Valcke, M., De Maeseneer, J., Derese, A., et al. Impact
of the transition from a conventional to an integrated contextual medical
curriculum on knowledge acquisition: a cross-sectional and longitudinal
approach. *Medical Education* 2008;43(7):704-13.

182 Dhaese, S.A.M., Van de Caveye, I., Vanden Bussche, P., Bogaert, S., De
Maeseneer, J. Student Participation: to the benefit of both the student
and the faculty. *Education for health* 2015;28(1). Available at: http://www.
educationforhealth.net/article.asp?issn=1357-6238;year=2015;volume=2
8;issue=1;spage=79;epage=82;aulast=Dhaese

183 IOM (Institute of Medicine). *Interprofessional Education for Collaboration:
learning how to improve health from interprofessional models across the
continuum of education to practice: workshop summary.* Washington, DC:
The National Academies Press, 2013.

184 Strategic Advisory Board Wellbeing, Health, Family. *Vision Statement:
New Professionalism in Care and Support as a Task for the Future.* Brussels,
Flemish Community, 17 December 2015. Available at: http://www.sarwgg.
be/sites/default/files/documenten/SARWGG_20151217_New%20
Professionalism_Vision%20statement_DEF.pdf

185 The Training for Health Equity Network. *THEnet's Social Accountability
Evaluation Framework version 1.* Monograph I (1 ed). The Training for
Health Equity Network, 2011. Available at: http://www.provost.utoronto.

ca/Assets/Provost+Digital+Assets/Provost/Provost+Digital+Assets/CHS/Training+For+Health+Equity+Network.pdf

186   IPEC. *Core Competencies for Interprofessional Collaborative Practice.* 2016. Available at: http://www.aacn.nche.edu/education-resources/IPEC-2016-Updated-Core-Competencies-Report.pdf

187   Available at: https://en.wikipedia.org/wiki/William_Osler

188   Pype, P. *Workplace Learning for General Practitioners in Palliative Care: Suitable and Feasible?* Doctoral thesis, Ghent University, 2014.

189   Fraser, S., Greenhalgh, R. Coping with complexity: educating for capability. *BMJ.* 2001;323(7316):799-803.

190   Obolensky, N. *Complex Adaptive Leadership.* Surrey, UK, Gower Publishing Limited, 2010.

191   Anderson, R., McDaniel, R. Managing health care organisations: where professionalism meets complexity science. *Health Care Manage Rev.* 2000;25(1):83-92.

192   De Sutter, A., van Driel, M., Maier, M., De Maeseneer, J. The new impact factor has arrived. Who cares? *European Journal of General Practice* 2015;21(3):153-4.

193   van Driel, M.L., Maier, M., De Maeseneer, J. Measuring the impact of family medicine research: scientific citations or societal impact? *Family Practice* 2007;24:401-2.

194   Ministry of the Flemish Community – Working Group Primary Health Care. *Horizontal Co-operation of the Care Disciplines in Primary Health Care.* Brussels, Ministry of the Flemish Community, 23rd of June 1983 (in Dutch, unpublished).

195   De Maeseneer, J., Aertgeerts, B., Remmen, R., Devroey, D. *Together We Change. Primary Health Care: Now More Than Ever!* Brussels, 9 December

Family Medicine and Primary Care

2014 (in Dutch) Available at: http://www.hapraktijkvoorbeelden.be/doc/together-we-change-ned.pdf

196 Anonymous. *Health 2020 : European Policy Framework and Strategy for the 21st Century.* Available at: http://www.euro.who.int/en/publications/policy-documents/health-2020.-a-european-policy-framework-and-strategy-for-the-21st-century-2013b

197 Scientific Institute for Public Health. *Health Survey 2013* (in Dutch). Available at: https://his.wiv-isp.be/NL/SitePages/Introductiepagina.aspx

198 Expert Panel on Effective Ways of Investing in Health (EXPH). *Access to health services in the European Union.* Brussels, EXPH, 30 May 2016. Available at: http://ec.europa.eu/health/expert_panel/sites/expertpanel/files/015_access_healthservices_en.pdf

199 Costa-Font, J., Rico, A. A vertical competition in the Spanish National Health System. *Public Choice* 2006;128(3-4):477-498.

200 World Health Organisation. *Strengthening the Model of Primary Health Care in Estonia. Assessment Report.* Copenhagen, WHO Regional Office for Europe, 2016. Available at: http://www.euro.who.int/__data/assets/pdf_file/0007/321946/Strengthening-model-primary-health-care-Estonia.PDF?ua=1

201 OECD. *Caring for Quality in Health: Lessons Learnt from 15 Reviews of Health Care Quality, OECD Reviews of Health Care Quality.* Paris, OECD Publishing, 2017. Available at: http://dx.doi.org/10.1787/9789264267787-en

202 Mickan, S.M. Evaluating the effectiveness of health care teams. Aust Health Rev 2005;29(2):2011-7.

203 WHO. *World Health Report: Primary Health Care, Now More Than Ever!* Geneva, World Health Organisation 2008. Available at: http://www.who.int/whr/2008/whr08_en.pdf

204 Kidd, M. *The Contribution of Family Medicine to Improving Health Systems: A Guidebook from the World Organisation of Family Doctors.* London, Radcliffe Publishing, 2013.

205 World Health Organisation. *World Health Report 2013: Research for Universal Health Coverage.* Geneva, WHO, 2013. Available at: http://apps. who.int/iris/bitstream/10665/85761/2/9789240690837_eng.pdf

206 World Health Organisation. *People-Centred and Integrated Health Services: An Overview of the Evidence.* Geneva, World Health Organisation, 2015. Available at: http://apps.who.int/iris/bitstream/10665/155004/1/WHO_ HIS_SDS_2015.7_eng.pdf?ua=1

207 *Primary Health Care Performance Initiative* (2015). Available at: http:// phcperformanceinitiative.org/

208 World Health Organisation – Regional Office for Europe. *The European Framework for Action on Integrated Health Services Delivery: An Overview.* Copenhagen, WHO Regional Office for Europe, 2016. Available at: http://www.euro.who.int/__data/assets/pdf_file/0010/317377/FFA-IHS-service-delivery-overview.pdf

209 Sixty-Second World Health Assembly. *Resolution WHA62.12. Primary health care, including health system strengthening.* May 22, 2009. Available at http://www.who.int/hrh/resources/A62_12_EN.pdf

210 Maarse, J., Jeurissen, P. The policy and politics of the 2015 long-term care reform in the Netherlands. *Health Policy* 2016;120(3):241-5.

211 Groenewegen, P., Heinemann, S., Greß, S., Schäfer, W. Primary Care practice composition in 34 countries. *Health Policy* 2015;119(2):1576-83.

212 Pavli, D.R., et al. Process quality indicators in family medicine: results of an international comparison. *BMC Family Practice* 2015;16:172.

213 De Maeseneer, J., Bogaerts, K., De Prins, L., Groenewegen, P. A Literature Review. In: Brown, S. *Physician Funding and Health Care Systems – An International Perspective. A summary of a conference hosted by the WHO,*

WONCA and RCGP at St-John's College, Cambridge. London, Royal College of General Practitioners, 1999, 17-31.

214 Annemans, L., Closon, M.C., Heymans, I., Lagasse, R., Mendes da Costa, E., et al. *Comparison of Cost and Quality of 2 Financing Systems for Primary Care in Belgium. Health Services Research (HSR)*. Brussels, Federal Knowledge Centre for Health Care (KCE); 2008. KCE report 85A (D/2008/10.273/49). Available at: https://kce.fgov.be/sites/default/files/page_documents/d20081027349_0.pdf

215 Expert Panel on Effective Ways of Investing in Health (EXPH). *Report on Access to Health Services in the European Union*. Brussels, European Union, 2016. Available at: http://ec.europa.eu/health/expert_panel/sites/expertpanel/files/015_access_healthservices_en.pdf

216 Scott, A., Sivey, P., Ait Ouakrim, D., Willenberg, L., Naccarilla, L., Furler, J., Young, D. The effect of financial incentives on the quality of health care provided by primary care physicians (review). *Cochrane database of systematic reviews* 2011, issue 9. Art. n°:CD008451.

217 Roland, M. Linking physicians' pay to the quality of care – a major experiment in the United Kingdom. *N Engl J Med* 2004;351:1448-54.

218 Healthcare Republic. *Independent Nurse QoF survey*. Available at: http://www.healthcarerepublic.com/news/GP/772416/Independent-Nurse-QoF-survey/

219 Campbell, S.M., McDonald, R., Lester, H. The experience of pay for performance in English family practice: a qualitative study. *Ann Fam Med* 2008;6(3):228-34.

220 Ryan, A.M., Krinsky, S., Kontopantelis, E., Doran, T. Long-term evidence for the effect of pay-for-performance in primary care on mortality in the UK: a population study. *Lancet* 2016;388:268-74. Available at: http://dx.doi.org/10.1016/S0140-6736(16)00276-2

221 van Loenen, T., van den Berg, M.J., Westert, G.P., Faber, M.J. Organisational aspects of primary care related to avoidable hospitalisation: a systematic review. *Family Practice*, 2014;31(5): 502-16.

222 van Loenen, T., Faber, M.J., Westert, G.P., van den Berg, M.J. The impact of primary care organisation on avoidable hospital admissions for diabetes in 23 countries. *Scand J Prim Health Care.* March, 2016;34(1):5-12.

223 De Maeseneer, J., De Prins, L., Gosset, C., Heyerick, J. Provider Continuity in Family Medicine: does it make a difference in total health care costs? *Ann Fam Med.* 2003;1:144-8.

224 Reibling, N., Wendt, C. *Regulating Patients' Access to Health Care Services. In: Merviö MM. Health Care Management and Economics: Perspectives on Public and Private Administration.* Hershey (USA), IGI Global, 2013, 53-68.

225 EXPH (Expert Panel on Effective Ways of Investing in Health). *Report on Definition of a frame of reference in relation to primary care with a special emphasis on financing systems and referral systems.* Brussels, 10 July 2014. Available at: http://ec.europa.eu/health/expert_panel/sites/expertpanel/files/004_definitionprimarycare_en.pdf

226 Robinson, R. User Chargers for Health Care. In: Mossialos E, Dixon A, Figueras J, Kutzin J (Eds.). *Funding Health Care: Options for Europe.* Milton Keynes, UK: Open University Press, 2002, 161-83.

227 Mossialos, E., Thomson, S. "Access to Health Care in the European Union: The Impact of User Charges and Voluntary Health Insurance." In: Gulliford, M., Morgan, M. (Eds.). *Access to health care.* London, UK, Routledge, 2003, 143-73.

228 OECD Health Policy Studies. *Better Ways to Pay for Health Care.* 2016, OECD Health Policy Studies, OECD Publishing, Paris. Available at: http://dx.doi.org/10.1787/9789264258211-en

229 Tsiachristas, A. Financial Incentives to Stimulate Integration of Care. *International Journal of Integrated Care*. 2016;16(4):8.

230 Anonymous. *Training in Family Medicine and Primary Health Care in South-Africa and Flanders: report of a study visit (16-25/09/97)*. Project number ZA.96.11, Minister of the Flemish Community, Department of Education.

231 Mash, R., Downing, R., Moosa, S., De Maeseneer, J. Exploring the key-principles of family medicine in sub-Saharan Africa: international Delphi-consensus process. *SA Fam Pract* 2008;50(3):60-5.

232 De Maeseneer, J., et al. Scaling up family medicine and primary health care in Africa: statement of the Primafamed-network, Victoria Falls, Zimbabwe. *Afr J Prim Health Care Fam Med*. 2013;5(1). Available at: http://dx.doi.org/10.4102/phcfm.v5i1.507

233 Khalid, G.M., Steinar, H., Samira, H.A., Elfatih, M.M. Scaling up Family Medicine training in Gezira, Sudan – a 2-year in-service master program using modern information and communication technology: a survey study. *Human Resources for Health* 2014;12:3. Available at: http://www.human-resources-health.com/content/12/1/3

234 Flinkenflögel, M., Essuman, A., Chege, P., Ayankogbe, O., De Maeseneer, J. Family Medicine Training in Sub-Saharan Africa: South-South co-operation in the Primafamed project as a strategy for development. *Fam Pract* 2014;31(4):427-36.

235 Tutu, D. *Preface: A Message of Hope. In: Hugo J, Allen L. Doctors of Tomorrow: Family Medicine in South-Africa*. Grahamstown NISC, VI-VII, 2008.

236 Anonymous. *Supporting Family Practice in Africa. European Commission, What Is Horizon 2020?* Available at: http://www.ec.europa.eu/programmes/horizon2020/en/news/supporting-family-practice-africa

237 Friends of Paul De Maeseneer. *A Voice for the Third World*. Ghent, Friends of Paul De Maeseneer, 1993.

238 Pankaj, M. "Welcome to the Age of Anger". *The Guardian*, 08 dec 2016. Available at: https://www.theguardian.com/politics/2016/dec/08/welcome-age-anger-brexit-trump

239 Davies, N. "Myanmar's Moment Of Truth." *The Guardian*. 09 mar 2016. Available at: https://www.theguardian.com/world/2016/mar/09/myanmar-moment-of-truth-aung-san-suu-kyi

240 Booth, R., Dodd, V., Parveen, N. "Labour MP Jo Cox Dies After Being Shot And Stabbed." *The Guardian*. 16 Jun 2016. Available at https://www.theguardian.com/uk-news/2016/jun/16/labour-mp-jo-cox-shot-in-west-yorkshire

241 Oxfam International. *An Economy for the 99%*. Oxfam International, 2017. Available at: https://www.oxfam.org/sites/www.oxfam.org/files/file_attachments/bp-economy-for-99-percent-160117-en.pdf

242 Szreter, S., Woolcock, M. Health by association? Social capital, social theory and a political economy of public health. *International Journal of Epidemiology* 2003;33:1-18.

243 WFPHA. A Global Charter for the Public's Health. *European Journal of Public Health*. 2016;26(2):210-2.

244 Starfield, B., Shi, L., Macinko, J. Contribution of Primary Care to Health Systems and Health. *The Milbank Quarterly* 2005;83(3):457-502.

245 Kringos, D.S., Boerma, W., van der Zee Groenewegen, P. Europe's strong primary care systems are linked to better population health but also to higher health spending. *Health Aff* 2013;32(4):686-694.

246 High-Level Commission on Health Employment and Economic Growth. *Working for Health and Growth: Investing in the Health Workforce*. Geneva, World Health Organization, 2016.

247 Pettigrew, L.M., De Maeseneer, J., Padula Anderson, M.-I., Essuman, E., Kidd, M.R., Haines A. Primary health care and the Sustainable Development Goals. *Lancet* 2015;386:2119-20.

248 Gillies, J.C.M., Mercer, S.W., Lyon, A., Scott, M., Watt, G.C.M. Distilling the essence of general practice: a learning journey in progress. *Br J Gen Pract* 2009;167-70.

249 Marmot, M. Post-truth and science. *Lancet* 2017;389:497-8.

250 Verlinde, E., Verdée, T., Van de Walle, M., Art, B., De Maeseneer, J., Willems, S. Unique health care utilisation patterns in a homeless population in Ghent. *BMC Health Services Research* 2010;10:242.

251 European Commission. *Communication from the Commission to the European Parliament, the Council, The European and Social Committee and the Committee of the Regions: Establishing a European Pillar of Social Rights.* Brussels, European Commission, 2017.

252 Horton, R. Off-line: science and the defeat of fear. *Lancet* 2017;389:1383.

253 Sanders, B. An agenda to fight inequality. *Lancet* 2017;389:1376-7.

254 Marmot, M. *Fair Society, Healthy Lives: The Marmot Review; Strategic Review of Health Inequalities in England post-2010*: [S.l.] : The Marmot Review; 2010.

255 Gilbran, K. *The Prophet.* 2010 (first published 1923). Kolkata: Rupa & Co.

What is the role of Primary Care in today's
and tomorrow's society?

How do we deal with an increase in health
inequality and the challenges of multi-morbidity?

How do we keep health care accessible
and sustainable in the future?

Modern family practices and Primary Care Centres are facing the challenges of increasing globalisation and migration. At the same time, a
culture of fear is hurting the principles of solidarity and social justice
on which health care systems are based. Practices, and in particular
the doctors and health professionals of tomorrow, are in need of a new
vision for the future.

Since the 1970s, Primary Care has become the cornerstone of health
care, with an all-important role for Family Medicine. *Family Medicine
and Primary Care* reviews this development, and puts it in perspective
against the backdrop of today's and tomorrow's fast-moving society.
Based on concrete testimonials and an analysis of case studies, this book
responds to the most urgent questions of today's family physicians.

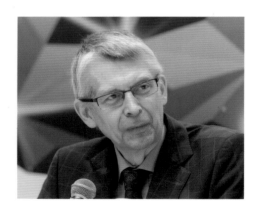

Jan De Maeseneer is Head of the
Department of Family Medicine and
Primary Health Care at Ghent Univer-
sity (1991-2017). From 2005 to 2017 he
was the Chairman of the European
Forum for Primary Care. In 2010 he was
appointed Director of the International
Centre for Primary Health Care and
Family Medicine-Ghent University, a
WHO Collaborating Centre on Primary
Health Care.

www.lannoocampus.com

9 789401 444460